Clinician's Guide to Common Drug Interactions in Primary Care

Eric Christianson, PharmD, BCPS, BCGP

Copyright and Disclaimer

Copyright © Eric Christianson 2019

ABOUT THE AUTHOR

Dr. Eric Christianson PharmD, BCPS, BCGP is a clinical pharmacist who is passionate about patient safety. Eric is the founder of meded101.com a website dedicated to providing quality, real world medication education for healthcare professionals. He has been quoted or acknowledged by The Wall Street Journal, American Journal of Nursing, Pharmacy Podcast, Pharmacy Today, and Pharmacy Times. He has authored Amazon Best Sellers such as *Pharmacotherapy; Clinical Pharmacy Pearls, Case Studies, and Common Sense* and *The Thrill of the Case*.

Eric is the creator of Real Life Pharmacology – A free podcast geared toward teaching healthcare students and young professionals about the critical medication pearls that will show up on board exams as well as in real life. The podcast is available at the website RealLifePharmacology.com as well as on iTunes. He also gives away a free 31 page PDF Pharmacology Study Guide of highly testable pearls on the top 200 drugs.

He is the principle author of popular webinars and study material for professional development as well as board certification exams (BCPS, NAPLEX, BCACP, BCGP and BCMTMS). You can find all of these resources at ***meded101.com/store***

Please take the time to check out the free resources provided through the website and social media accounts.

Real Life Pharmacology (Free Top 200 Study Guide) –
RealLifePharmacology.com

Subscribers to the Meded101.com Blog; Free 6 page PDF –
30 Medication Mistakes

Facebook – Meded101

Twitter - @mededucation101

LinkedIn – Eric Christianson, PharmD BCGP, BCPS

Nursing Facebook Page – NCLEX Pharmacology

Pharmacists and Healthcare Students may also be interested in Board Exam Prep Material and other clinical pharmacy resources:
@ **Meded101.com/store**
- BCPS
- NAPLEX
- BCACP
- BCGP
- BCMTMS
- NCLEX
- And More!

INTRODUCTION

For many, drug interactions are one of the most frustrating challenges in primary care, geriatrics, and ambulatory care practice. Even if one is up to speed on what drugs interact with one another, it is often unknown how to manage that specific interaction. Throughout the book, I share some of my management tips and pearls to help you feel more comfortable in managing drug interactions.

This book is a perfect piece of education for pharmacists, nurse practitioners, physicians, physician assistants, and nurses who are looking to pick up clinical, real world practice pearls.

Table of Contents

Chapter 1: Mechanisms of Drug Interactions

Drug interactions can present some of the most difficult challenges to a growing clinician. In this book, I am going to talk about some of the most common drug interactions and hopefully help provide some insight on the seriousness of those interactions. In addition, my goal is to teach you strategies to manage some of these drug interactions. All drug interactions are not created equal. Some drug interactions can be managed by monitoring and some drug interactions you should avoid. You'll need a basic understanding of drug interactions and how they occur. This introductory chapter will give you a nice background on how drug interactions occur. Here's a breakdown of how some of the most common drug interactions occur.

Additive Effects

Medications have similar side effect profiles. When it comes to drug interactions, adding another medication that can cause an adverse effect similar to a medication our patient is already taking can be problematic. Here's a couple of common examples to demonstrate this risk.

Example 1

AU is a 78 year old female with a history of hypertension, edema, GERD, diabetes, and neuropathy. She is currently taking amlodipine 10 mg daily, hydrochlorothiazide 12.5 mg daily, omeprazole 20 mg daily, aspirin 81 mg daily, and metformin 500 mg twice daily. She would like to have a medication to help with her troublesome peripheral neuropathy. Pregabalin 50 mg three times per day is added to her regimen.

Within a week of this addition, she begins to experience pitting edema and is placed on furosemide 40 mg daily for 5 days. The pregabalin alone can cause this side effect and in this case, that may be the most consequential factor. It should not go unnoticed, however, that amlodipine is a very common cause of peripheral edema. Recognizing this cumulative risk is important to remember in situations where the timing of the onset of edema or another adverse effect is not so pronounced.

Example 2

Let's take a look at AU in another situation. She is currently receiving the same medications as mentioned before. As a reminder, her medication list includes amlodipine 10 mg daily, hydrochlorothiazide 12.5 mg daily, omeprazole 20 mg daily, aspirin 81 mg daily, and metformin 500 mg twice daily.

We find out that her diabetes is out of control. She has an A1C of 10.2 and we determine that we'd like to add an SGLT-2 inhibitor to her regimen. The SGLT-2 inhibitors like empagliflozin, dapagliflozin, and canagliflozin are unique in how they help lower blood sugars. The SGLT-2 inhibitors reduce blood sugar by increasing the output of blood glucose through the urine. In the transport of glucose out through the kidney and into the urine, water can also go with it. In this patient case, the hydrochlorothiazide will also have a diuretic effect. The risk of this additive effect could lead to a reduction in blood volume. With a reduction in blood volume, there is a risk for volume depletion, dehydration, and lower blood pressure.

In patients who are on other medications that can contribute to volume depletion and hypotension, an SGLT-2 has the potential to compound this effect. Another risk of volume depletion is that it may increase the risk of acute renal failure through dehydration. Monitoring for dizziness, checking lab work like renal function, and assessing blood pressure would be critical when considering adding an SGLT-2 to a patient already taking a diuretic.

Opposing Effects

Example 1

Many drugs will work on various receptors throughout the body. To use as an educational point, there is no better example to point to than the beta receptor. Beta-blockers are frequently used in clinical practice for their ability to lower blood pressure and slow the heart rate. Both of these beneficial actions are primarily achieved by blocking the effects of beta-1 receptors.

All beta-blockers are not created equally. Some beta-blockers have action on alternative beta receptors. Propranolol is one such beta-blocker that is classified as a non-selective beta-blocker. This means that in addition to the positive effects on beta-1 receptors, it can also have blocking effects on beta-2 receptors.

Activation of beta-2 receptors can help improve a patient's breathing by relaxing the smooth muscles of the respiratory tract. In patients with asthma and COPD, this activation of beta-2 receptors can be life-changing. The blockade of the beta-2 receptor by propranolol can also be life-changing. It can directly oppose beta-2 agonists like albuterol from having their beneficial effects of opening up the airway.

Example 2

Metoclopramide can be used for various GI symptoms like gastroparesis and nausea. One of the primary parts of this drug's mechanism of action is that it can block dopamine receptors.

Dopamine plays a critical role in the pathogenesis of Parkinson's disease. In a patient with Parkinson's, it is well recognized that these patients have a deficiency of dopamine in the brain. Because of this, we try to supplement the body with extra dopamine to help manage some of the motor complications due to the lack of dopamine.

When we add a drug like metoclopramide to a patient's medication regimen, we have created a situation where the effect of dopamine can be blunted. This can lead to an increase in the likelihood of Parkinson's symptoms reoccurring.

In a similar fashion, excessive dopamine can induce nausea and vomiting. With the use of metoclopramide, this may be exactly the symptoms that we are trying to manage. It is critical to recognize how drugs work and what adverse effects that they cause so we are not overusing medications to treat conditions that are caused by a medication with opposing effects.

Enzyme Inhibition

Example 1

Medication metabolism is arguably the largest and most clinically significant source for drug interactions. Medications that are primarily metabolized by enzymes in the liver can be greatly affected if we affect how those enzymes work. CYP3A4 is one of the most well studied and well-known enzymes that can impact hundreds to maybe even thousands of drugs.

Apixaban is an oral anticoagulant that is broken down at least in part by CYP3A4. By using a CYP3A4 inhibitor like erythromycin, there is the potential to raise concentrations of apixaban. This could lead to a higher risk of bleeding.

Example 2

Another less common example that will be discussed further in the book is CYP2C8. Gemfibrozil is a medication that can inhibit the activity of this enzyme. If a drug is significantly broken down by CYP2C8 and the patient is taking gemfibrozil, there will be a higher likelihood of elevated concentrations of that drug. Pioglitazone is an example of a medication that can have its concentrations raised by gemfibrozil.

Being aware of some of the signs and symptoms of pioglitazone's adverse effect profile would be critical to assessing and managing the risk of this drug interaction.

Enzyme Induction

Example 1

Carbamazepine is a drug that you must know. This drug is a potent enzyme inducer. This differs significantly from an enzyme inhibitor and will have the exact opposite clinical effect. Drugs that are inactivated by liver enzymes will be inactivated more quickly in a patient taking an enzyme inducer. Going back to our prior apixaban example above, carbamazepine can induce CYP3A4 and facilitate a more efficient and swifter breakdown of the drug. Bleeding will be less likely. The risk for treatment failure, usually in the form of a blood clot, will be more likely.

Example 2

MW is a 19 year old female with a history of well-controlled seizures. She has historically taken phenytoin without any concerns. She begins to take oral contraceptives to prevent pregnancy. This is likely going to be a scary interaction to try to deal with. Because of the ability of phenytoin to induce the enzymes that breakdown estrogen and progesterone, it can significantly impair the ability of birth control to prevent pregnancy.

Alteration in Absorption

Binding interactions can be consequential. Many medications have the potential to bind one another in the gut. This can lead to lower concentrations of a specific medication. Calcium and iron are two of the most common examples of medications that can bind other drugs.

Many antibiotics like quinolones and tetracyclines can have their absorption significantly reduced because of binding interactions. There are a few common ways to deal with this interaction. One of the methods would be to hold or discontinue the agent that is binding up the antibiotic. Another potential option is to try to schedule the doses as far away from one another as possible. For example, if a patient is to take levofloxacin in the morning for 5 days, they could take their calcium in the evening.

Absorption drug interactions are usually fairly easy to manage when identified. One of the greatest challenges with this drug interaction is recognizing it at the onset of therapy initiation. An experienced, skilled clinician will hopefully recognize the risk associated with this interaction and time the medications appropriately or avoid the interaction altogether.

Alteration in Protein Binding

By remembering that unbound drug is an active drug, you should appreciate the risk for protein binding alterations. A significant number of medications can bind proteins in the bloodstream. As this occurs, that drug is not freely available to create physiologic effects. When another medication is added that can also bind these proteins, this can displace other medications and increase the quantity of free drug in the bloodstream. This essentially allows for enhanced physiologic effects.

Warfarin is a medication that is highly protein-bound. When another drug is added that can kick warfarin off of those protein binding sites, it can free up warfarin which will increase the likelihood of elevating the patient's INR and increase their bleed risk.

Alteration in Renal Elimination

Some drugs can alter the way other medications are eliminated through the kidney. Chlorthalidone, like all thiazide diuretics, has the potential to block the excretion of lithium from the kidney. This can lead to lithium toxicity.

This type of interaction, while significant, is much less common than drug interactions involving the liver and CYP enzyme pathways.

16

P-glycoprotein is a protein found in many cell membranes in the body and essentially acts as a pump. P-glycoprotein can pump drugs across cell membranes. This can alter drug concentrations and ultimately efficacy and safety.

P-glycoprotein is useful to the body as it can help pump toxins out of the body and out of individual cells. For many medications, the body is going to treat it similar to any toxin. Our patients are often clinically impacted by P-glycoprotein found in the gut. Its action in the gut serves to pump toxins or drugs back into the gut lumen for elimination out of the body. The action of P-glycoprotein in the gut can serve to reduce drug concentrations. Medications like the non-dihydropyridine calcium channel blockers can inhibit the action of P-glycoprotein. This can lead to higher concentrations of medications that are typically (at least in part) removed from the body through this mechanism.

In part because of its P-glycoprotein inhibition, there is potential that a drug like verapamil could raise concentrations of anticoagulants like apixaban and rivaroxaban. Monitoring for the risk of bleeding due to higher anticoagulant concentrations would be appropriate in this situation.

Renal Failure Risk

There is always a huge challenge in navigating CHF and CKD in our patients. The use of diuretics with ACE inhibitors can be life-altering in a very good way for patients who have fluid overload. The difficulty lies in keeping adequate perfusion to the kidney. Let's review a case scenario.

A 69 year old male presents to the emergency department with increasing shortness of breath. He has a very high pro-BNP which is indicative of the diagnosis of acute heart failure. In addition, he also has a substantially reduced ejection fraction. Prior to hospitalization, he reports that he has been out of the house the previous few days so he didn't want to take his furosemide because it makes him have to go to the bathroom all day. This change in adherence likely precipitated the heart failure exacerbation.

In the hospital, he has been receiving furosemide and is discharged on 40 mg twice daily. In addition, he also had an increase in his lisinopril to 20 mg per day.

At 2 weeks post-hospital checkup, the patient reports that he has had some significant shoulder pain from an old injury. He has been taking ibuprofen 800 mg three times per day. Upon assessment of his labs, his creatinine has risen from 1.2 to 2.8.

The increase in the diuretic, lisinopril, and the patient adding to the problem by taking the ibuprofen all potentially added to the worsening kidney function. The lisinopril and diuretic are incredibly important medications for heart failure, but we have to recognize the potential for kidney impairment.

When specifically looking at the physiology of this interaction, hopefully, you'll understand why this combination can cause renal failure. The glomerulus is critical to the function of the kidney. It essentially acts as a filter. To be functional, the glomerulus needs to have adequate pressure. The afferent arteriole is the blood vessel providing blood flow to the glomerulus. The efferent arteriole is the vessel that takes the blood away from the glomerulus and back towards the heart. NSAIDs, like ibuprofen, can cause the afferent arteriole to constrict. The ACE inhibitors and ARBs work on the backside of the glomerulus and can prevent vasoconstriction. This dysregulation can cause the glomerulus to lose control of the pressure it needs to maintain to effectively do its job of filtration.

The use of diuretics in combination with an ACE inhibitor and NSAID can compound this problem by further lowering the pressure in the vessels by removing fluid out of the arterioles. This is the process by which this combination of drugs can cause renal failure. You may hear this referred to more specifically as prerenal failure which indicates that hypoperfusion (or loss of blood flow) to the kidney has caused renal failure.

Managing the balance of protecting the kidney and adequately treating symptoms of heart failure is a big challenge. The first action in the case of acute renal failure caused by this triple combination would be to find an alternative analgesic to the ibuprofen that isn't going to hurt the kidney. Returning the kidney to normal function would certainly trump any analgesic benefit of the ibuprofen for his shoulder pain.

Following this action, the diuretic and ACE inhibitor doses would need to be looked at and potentially reduced. If the fluid status was much improved with the diuretic being on board for several days, then reducing the diuretic would make a lot of sense. Continued monitoring of the renal function to ensure that the GFR was going back up to baseline would be absolutely essential in monitoring this drug interaction.

Potassium Elevating Drugs

With a huge role in the management of hypertension, ACE inhibitors and ARBs will likely be the most common medication in your practice that can cause hyperkalemia. From a mechanism of action standpoint, the downstream effects of ACE Inhibitors and ARBs leads to a reduction in aldosterone. Aldosterone plays an important role in the function of the kidney by causing potassium excretion. By having less aldosterone, it leads to reduced excretion and potentially hyperkalemia. There are numerous other drugs that can interact with ACE inhibitors and ARBs to enhance the hyperkalemia risk. Here are a few common ones to look out for.

Aldosterone Antagonists

Aldosterone antagonists play a significant role in managing hypertension and are also a class of drugs that can be used to help with edema, ascites, and heart failure. Use is common and this class can also be commonly used in combination with ACE Inhibitors or ARBs. While there can be significant benefits from concomitant use, using these drugs in combination can strongly increase the risk of hyperkalemia.

Potassium Supplements

It may seem obvious to point out, but potassium supplements can raise potassium levels. I wanted to specifically mention this because I have seen patients use supplements on their own without it being listed on their medication list. It is critical to ask about supplements. On rare occasions, I have also seen this missed on medication reconciliation. The most common situation where I've seen potassium supplements cause hyperkalemia is where a patient stops taking a loop or thiazide diuretic and continues to take their prescribed supplement.

Trimethoprim

Trimethoprim is an antibiotic, most often used in combination with sulfamethoxazole. This drug is well-known to cause hyperkalemia. Here's a case scenario on this drug interaction.

JS is an 88 year old female who was recently diagnosed with a urinary tract infection. About 6 days ago, she had been started on sulfamethoxazole/trimethoprim for a period of 10 days. Other medications include:
- Spironolactone
- Metformin
- Rosuvastatin
- Valsartan
- Carvedilol
- Aspirin
- Amlodipine

This patient was a resident of a long term care facility and happened to be due for her twice yearly BMP. The majority of labs were stable with previous results. The potassium was substantially increased. The potassium level 6 months ago was 4.9 mEq/L and the potassium level today was 6.4. The patient was asymptomatic.

The use of spironolactone and valsartan would be contributing factors to the elevation in potassium. In addition to those two medications, trimethoprim likely compounded the risk of hyperkalemia.

Since this was on day 6 of treatment and the symptoms had completely resolved, the attending provider decided to stop the sulfamethoxazole/trimethoprim and hold the spironolactone with a potassium recheck tomorrow and increased monitoring of blood pressure.

In this case, it would have been interesting to look back at spironolactone and valsartan to see if these doses have been consistent over the previous 6 months. In addition to this, patient adherence should also be assessed although this would be less likely to be problematic given the patient likely receives her medication from the long term care facility.

Trimethoprim is purported to mechanistically act similar to the potassium-sparing diuretic amiloride in its ability to contribute to hyperkalemia. It can ultimately reduce the ability of the kidney to eliminate potassium from the body.

Amiloride

This potassium-sparing diuretic is not used to a great extent anymore, but can be a potential contributor to hyperkalemia if used in combination with an ACE inhibitor or ARB. Amiloride antagonizes sodium channels in the distal convoluted tubule (DCT) and collecting duct which inhibits sodium reabsorption. Because of this action and an alteration in sodium concentrations, this slows the activity of Na+/K+ATPase which can ultimately lead to higher potassium concentrations in the blood.

Heparin

Heparin can also have some aldosterone suppressing activity. The extent and frequency of hyperkalemia are likely going to be less than with ACE inhibitors, ARBs, and aldosterone antagonists, but it is worth it to mention this drug. Keep an extra close eye on those patients who may already be at risk for hyperkalemia (i.e. renal disease or concomitant drugs that cause hyperkalemia).

Managing Hyperkalemia Interactions

I have seen inappropriate changes when it comes to this interaction. Sometimes inexperience clinicians, nurses, pharmacists may think that if there is a drug interaction, you automatically have to stop or change the interacting medication. While this can be true of some medications that are contraindicated when used together, this is not the case with the above-mentioned interactions concerning potassium.

The primary action one should take is to review the potassium level at baseline and following the initiation of the drugs. A clinician should be extra careful in a few common situations. If a patient is already hyperkalemic, you could understand how it would be problematic placing a patient on another medication or combination of medications that could enhance the hyperkalemia risk.

Another situation to proceed cautiously is when using interacting medications that cause hyperkalemia is when the patient has significant renal disease. The kidney is critical to eliminating potassium from the body and maintaining electrolyte balance. Any damage to the kidney can exacerbate the risk from medications that can cause hyperkalemia.

Lithium

ACE inhibitors and Angiotensin Receptor Blockers (ARBs) are incredibly common for the management of hypertension. Because they generally don't have a ton of drug interactions compared to other agents, they may be overlooked by a prescribing provider. ACE inhibitors and ARBs can significantly raise the concentrations of lithium, potentially leading to toxicity.

There are a few strategies to consider when addressing the interaction with lithium. The easiest and most obvious strategy is to monitor the patient. With the good possibility of lithium concentrations increasing, some signs of toxicity to monitor include: CNS changes like confusion, ataxia, GI upset, and tremor.

If we employ another strategy, we could consider changing medications. We likely are not going to change the lithium as many patients with bipolar disorder are likely going to benefit and need this medication long term. We are likely going to look at changing the ACE or ARB. Since we have so many alternative medications to help manage hypertension, this would be the best course to avoid the interaction altogether. Reviewing the past medical history and what has been tried for hypertension would be critical. Alternative antihypertensives might include calcium channel blockers like amlodipine or a beta-blocker like metoprolol. Thiazide diuretics can also interact with lithium by raising drug concentrations, so avoidance of this class of antihypertensive as an alternative would be important if we are trying to avoid more drug interactions.

Lastly, if the ACE inhibitor or ARB is felt to be appropriate and there is no desire to change lithium, we would want to closely monitor lithium levels and adjust the lithium dose as appropriate.

Blood Pressure Lower Agents

ACE Inhibitors and ARBs are routinely used for blood pressure lowering effects. This can be an excellent benefit that can reduce the risk of renal disease, cardiovascular events and many other negative health outcomes due to hypertension. This may be a little obvious, but you do have to be a little extra cautious in patients who are already receiving other agents that can cause orthostasis. Most obvious, other antihypertensives like beta-blockers, diuretics, and calcium channel blockers can increase this risk. In addition to these agents that are commonly used for their blood pressure lowering effects, there are other medications that can cause orthostasis despite not having a primary indication for hypertension. Common examples of other medications that may exacerbate orthostasis include carbidopa/levodopa, antipsychotics, trazodone, PDE-5 inhibitors for erectile dysfunction like sildenafil and tadalafil, and dopamine agonists like pramipexole and ropinirole. I won't discuss this much further, but all blood pressure-lowering agents will carry the risk of bringing down the blood pressure too much and causing orthostatic hypotension.

Blood Pressure Increasing Agents

While NSAIDs can significantly increase the risk of renal impairment when combined with ACE Inhibitors, it is important to note that NSAIDs can cause vasoconstriction that also oppose the blood pressure lowering effects of ACE inhibitors. Any type of stimulant use must also be monitored for its potential to oppose the antihypertensive nature of ACE Inhibitors and ARBs.

Angioedema Risk

I always emphasize to healthcare students that you must understand or look up brand name medications if you are unsure of the components of that medication. There is no better example of this than the drug Entresto. Entresto (sacubitril/valsartan) is a brand name medication that can be used in the management of heart failure. The risk of using

Entresto with another ACE Inhibitor is angioedema. This is absolutely a contraindication. This combination should not be used together. Entresto requires a 36 hour washout period when switching from one to the other.

Dihydropyridine Calcium Channel Blockers

Calcium channel blockers are used for a variety of indications and are commonly found in clinical practice. Let's start with a case scenario regarding the amlodipine and simvastatin interaction.

Amlodipine Simvastatin

A 64 year old female is taking the following medications:
- Alendronate 70 mg weekly
- Amlodipine 10 mg daily
- Folic acid 1 mg twice daily
- Furosemide 20 mg daily
- Gabapentin 300 mg BID
- Humalog 5 units with meals
- Lansoprazole 30 mg daily
- Insulin glargine 10 units twice daily
- Losartan 100 mg daily
- Metoprolol 100 mg BID
- Oxycodone 5 mg three times daily
- Pramipexole 0.25 mg at bedtime
- Sertraline 100 mg daily
- Simvastatin 40 mg at bedtime
- Sumatriptan 50 mg as needed for migraines
- Solifenacin 5 mg daily

In this case scenario, we will attempt to address the amlodipine simvastatin interaction. Currently, the FDA recommends a max dose of simvastatin 20 mg daily if a patient is also receiving amlodipine. The major concern with this drug interaction is an elevation in simvastatin concentration which could contribute to the risk of rhabdomyolysis. There are a few things to consider when trying to come up with a solution to manage this interaction.

When assessing what to do about this drug interaction, the first item I would look at is the cardiovascular risk. By the medication list, we are going to assume that this patient has a medical history of diabetes. This would certainly place her at some level of cardiovascular risk

24

which may necessitate a higher intensity statin right now, or possibly in the future.

Before considering any medication changes, reviewing a drug allergy and intolerance list is not something you should overlook. This is something that I have been personally burned by and have also seen many others look bad by suggesting or changing to a medication that a patient previously did not tolerate.

A further cardiovascular assessment would need to be done, but due to the likelihood she is at higher cardiovascular risk, I'd lean towards changing the simvastatin to a higher intensity statin like atorvastatin or rosuvastatin.

Changing the amlodipine in this situation is less desirable to me. This is especially true if the blood pressure is under good control. In looking at the dosages of some of the other antihypertensive medications like losartan and metoprolol, we don't have a lot of room to increase those medications if we discontinue the amlodipine.

Another option is to leave it alone. I have seen some clinicians do this if the patient has been on the combination for a long time without issue. It isn't my ideal choice. If this patient begins to take another medication that interacts with simvastatin (examples include amiodarone, grapefruit juice, certain macrolide antibiotics or HIV medications, this could really cause simvastatin concentrations to go through the roof. A substantial risk for rhabdomyolysis would happen as a result of this. Drugs that inhibit the CYP3A4 enzyme would be of high concern for their ability to raise concentrations of simvastatin in addition to the amlodipine.

Opposition of Antihypertensive Effect

Drug-induced resistant hypertension does happen. It is important to recognize medications that can contribute to this as well as recognize when patients are on higher doses of these medications that may elevate blood pressure. Here's the scenario:
A 62 y/o female has a past medical history of:
- CHF
- HTN
- GERD
- OA
- Neuropathy
- Recent BP = 168/78

Medication list:
- Lasix 20 mg daily
- Celebrex 200 mg BID
- Lisinopril 40 mg daily
- Amlodipine 10 mg daily
- Effexor XR 300 mg daily
- Metoprolol tartrate 100 mg BID
- Ibuprofen 400 mg PRN
- Omeprazole 20 mg daily
- Aspirin 81 mg daily
- Lipitor 10 mg daily

She has tried numerous medications for blood pressure and is still consistently above 160 systolic. The amlodipine in combination with lisinopril and metoprolol has not been effective at reducing the patient's blood pressure.

In this situation, I would certainly be looking at the duplication in using celecoxib and ibuprofen. Assessment of the as needed dose of ibuprofen and how much they are using it would be important. A thorough workup of pain and identification of medications tried in the past would be important. If it hasn't been tried, acetaminophen would be an option as well as topical analgesics if the OA is localized.

If neuropathic pain is more problematic, certainly we could look further at some of the antiseizure (but would need to be careful with pregabalin and gabapentin with potential to impact CHF) medications.

The other medication that I would be looking at in regards to possible drug-induced resistant hypertension would be the venlafaxine. While at lower doses, this medication does not tend to contribute to this problem, higher doses can possibly contribute to hypertension. Timing is always important in these scenarios as well. If this had been added/increased recently that would lead me even more down the path of trying to reduce this medication.

Azole Antifungals

Azole antifungals (fluconazole, ketoconazole, etc.) can raise the concentration of amlodipine. The end result of this potential interaction is going to be an increased risk for lower blood pressure and adverse effects from amlodipine.

Monitoring and educating the patient about the risk of low blood pressure and dizziness could be part of the strategy to manage this interaction. Elevated amlodipine concentrations could also cause a higher risk of toxicity in the form of edema or constipation.

Depending upon the indication the azole antifungal is being use for, another solution would be to try to find a different antifungal agent that would avoid this interaction.

In the event of clinically significant risk to the patient due to higher concentrations of amlodipine, a dose reduction of amlodipine would be a reasonable option. It is important to remember that when the antifungal is discontinued, the patient will likely have to resume the previous dose of amlodipine that their blood pressure was controlled on.

Calcium Channel Blockers and Phenytoin

There are numerous agents within this class of medication that can contribute to increased phenytoin concentrations (amlodipine, nifedipine, diltiazem, verapamil, etc.). This can ultimately cause toxicity in our patients on chronic phenytoin. This is particularly troublesome as phenytoin has a narrow therapeutic index. This essentially means that even small elevations in phenytoin concentrations could lead to toxicity. Monitoring patients for signs of phenytoin toxicity and assessing drug levels would be very important. It would be very unlikely that you would ever discontinue or change the phenytoin to a different medication due to this drug interaction, but it might be reasonable to consider another antihypertensive medication if alternatives exist. Based upon any changes in drug levels or signs of toxicity, one would also likely consider a reduction in phenytoin dosing with careful memory that phenytoin has very unique pharmacokinetics.

It is challenging to label this as a class effect. Recognize that drugs within the calcium channel blocker class may interact with phenytoin to varying degrees. A stronger interaction may exist with nifedipine while amlodipine may be less likely to cause a significant reaction.

Cumulative Adverse Effects

When we are using calcium channel blockers, one really important adverse effect to consider is edema. I do review the medication list to identify patients who may be at risk for edema. There are numerous medications that can induce edema and/or exacerbate heart failure symptoms. Some of the common medications I look out for cumulative edema side effects include NSAIDs, pioglitazone, and the gabapentinoids like pregabalin and gabapentin.

Non-Dihydropyridine Calcium Channel Blockers (Diltiazem and Verapamil)

CYP3A4 Inhibition

Diltiazem inhibits the enzyme CYP3A4 to an appreciable extent. When you think of drug interactions and a medication that can impact CYP3A4, you must recognize that this can impact numerous medications. Some of the medications that diltiazem interacts with include colchicine, tacrolimus, cyclosporine, cilostazol, warfarin, fentanyl, phenytoin, simvastatin, atorvastatin, and many HIV medications.

Verapamil is the other commonly used non-dihydropyridine. It has an overlapping drug interaction profile with diltiazem and can cause many of the same CYP3A4 drug interactions that diltiazem can. By inhibiting CYP3A4, these drugs are going to raise the concentrations of drugs that are metabolically broken down by CYP3A4.

In general, when comparing diltiazem and verapamil to the more commonly used amlodipine, it is critical to remember these drugs will have more drug interactions and likely more clinically significant drug interactions. This is primarily due to verapamil and diltiazem's impact on the CYP3A4 enzyme.

P-glycoprotein Inhibition

In addition to activity on CYP3A4, the non-dihydropyridine calcium channel blockers also have activity on P-glycoprotein. This protein is found in many cell membranes in the body and essentially acts as a pump. P-glycoprotein can pump drugs across cell membranes. This can alter drug concentrations and ultimately efficacy.

More specifically, this drug class inhibits P-glycoprotein and limits the efflux of certain medications out of the body. This can lead to higher concentrations of medications that are typically (at least in part) removed from the body through this mechanism.

In part because of its P-glycoprotein inhibition, there is potential that a drug like verapamil could raise concentrations of anticoagulants like apixaban and rivaroxaban. At a minimum, clinical monitoring of the patient could be done. Monitoring hemoglobin and educating the patient to be aware of bleeding and bruising would be appropriate.

In addition to the non-dihydropyridine calcium channel blockers, common agents like amiodarone, macrolides, some azole antifungals, and carvedilol can have the potential for inhibitory effects on P-glycoprotein.

Trazodone Diltiazem

A 74 year old patient was recently diagnosed with atrial fibrillation. Rate control was the preferred method of management by cardiology, but unfortunately, beta-blockers were not tolerable in this patient.

Diltiazem was initiated to help improve tachycardia and manage atrial fibrillation. It worked well, and vital signs were well maintained. Pulses were in the 60-70 range and blood pressure was fine with no indication of orthostasis symptoms.

Within a week of beginning to take the diltiazem, the patient did report that she was more fatigued. She felt as if she could "sleep all day". Diltiazem itself could certainly be responsible for this adverse effect. What was also of note is that she was on trazodone 100 mg at bedtime for insomnia. Diltiazem is a well-known CYP3A4 inhibitor. Any medication that is broken down by this enzyme can have its concentrations rise if we inhibit this enzyme. Trazodone is one of those medications.

With the addition of diltiazem, this likely increased the concentrations of trazodone. One of the most common adverse effects of trazodone is sedation. With the higher concentrations, we are more likely to have made this patient sleepier. I did mention that the diltiazem could do this as well and that has to be a consideration.

As a clinician, it is critical to do the best we can to provide a solution. In this case, the patient is well controlled with the new diltiazem Rx. I would be reluctant to switch this to another agent for atrial fibrillation. The simplest solution would be to titrate the dose of trazodone in a downward fashion and try to minimize the risk of sedation due to likely increased concentrations from the trazodone diltiazem interaction.

Diltiazem Donepezil Interaction – Cumulative Effects

Acetylcholinesterase Inhibitors are used in various forms of dementia. They can provide some symptom improvement in dementia, but cannot reverse or stop its progression. We need to remember that the agents aren't without risk. Here's a case to remember with acetylcholinesterase inhibitors and bradycardia.

An 82 year old male with mild Alzheimer's dementia has had some worsening symptoms of memory loss. He has a past history of MI, Raynaud's disorder, and kidney disease.

Current vitals:
- BP – 138/72
- Pulse – 54

Current medications include:
- Aspirin 81 mg daily
- Diltiazem XR 240 mg once daily
- Ranitidine 150 mg as needed for heartburn
- Lisinopril 5 mg daily

Family and the PCP would like to begin treatment with donepezil. Donepezil 10 mg once daily is initiated. Following initiation, he did not report any GI complaints. GI complaints are usually the most common adverse effect of the acetylcholinesterase inhibitors. Drug-induced weight loss is also a possible adverse effect. A drop in heartrate has a much lower rate of occurrence but can occur.

The family did notice increased lethargy and upon reassessment of the vital signs, the pulse was now 46. The diltiazem dose had remained consistent and there were no other changes. This was likely a worsening of bradycardia due to the donepezil. The starting dose was also inappropriately aggressive.

The best way I remember the acetylcholinesterase inhibitors and bradycardia reaction, is to recognize that anticholinergics (atropine) is used to treat bradycardia. Acetylcholinesterase inhibitors do the exact opposite of atropine as we saw in this case scenario.

There's a couple of options that I would consider in this situation. Depending upon the indication and clinical response, reducing the dose of diltiazem is a reasonable option. Another possibility is to assess the risk of continuing with donepezil. If the indication is there for this patient, discontinuation might be a consideration in favor of memantine. Memantine works differently than donepezil and would be very unlikely to have any impact on the heart.

Another option would be to go without the donepezil altogether. Given similar mechanisms of action, switching to another acetylcholinesterase inhibitor (i.e. rivastigmine) likely wouldn't be a viable choice to avoid bradycardia.

Verapamil/Phenytoin Interaction

JS is 38 year old male who has been on phenytoin for seizure prophylaxis for several years. He reports to his primary care provider complaining of severe headaches. He is diagnosed with cluster headaches. Over the next year, he continues to have period attacks and is placed on verapamil for cluster headache prophylaxis.

The verapamil and phenytoin interaction is a bit more complex than most drug interactions. The phenytoin affects the verapamil and the verapamil can affect the phenytoin. More specifically, the phenytoin is a notorious enzyme inducer. By inducing the enzyme that is primarily responsible for breaking down the verapamil, it can reduce concentrations. Verapamil will likely have reduced concentrations and there will be more opportunity for treatment failure of the cluster headaches

On the flipside, verapamil can inhibit CYP3A4. CYP3A4 is partly responsible for the metabolic breakdown of phenytoin. Phenytoin concentrations would likely rise on account of this interaction. We would want to assess levels prior to initiating the verapamil. If that phenytoin level is at the upper limit of normal, you should be a little more concerned. Once started, we'd encourage the patient to monitor for signs of phenytoin toxicity.

Sedation, ataxia, slurred speech, confusion, and GI upset are some common signs of phenytoin toxicity. Another good opportunity to monitor this interaction would be to assess follow up phenytoin levels within a week or two of making this change. Starting at a very low dose would also be a way to try to gently approach this combination if avoiding the combination is not possible.

Opposing Action

Epinephrine is the mainstay of therapy in a patient who is having a severe allergic reaction. Epinephrine has both alpha and beta receptor activity. By stimulating beta-2 receptors, we can cause smooth muscle relaxation in the lungs which allows a patient to breathe easier. The heart is also stimulated by beta-1 receptor activation. But what if these patients are on beta-blockers?

There is the potential that a beta-blocker will prevent the beneficial cardiac and respiratory impacts of epinephrine in the setting of an allergic reaction. This is not considered a contraindication and epinephrine will remain the drug of choice, but in the event a patient has a history of not responding well to epinephrine, this reason might be considered and attempting to mitigate this interaction might be appropriate.

There is some evidence that glucagon can be utilized in patients who have an anaphylaxis episode that is not relieved by epinephrine.

Beta-blockers can blunt the effect of albuterol. The extent of this interaction can depend upon multiple factors. The dose of the beta-blocker as well as the selectivity of the beta-blocker are two essential factors that may increase the risk for this interaction. Non-selective agents like propranolol have a much greater potential to create a significant drug interaction with albuterol because non-selective agents will inhibit beta-2 receptors. I discuss this further in the respiratory section.

Propranolol Ciprofloxacin Interaction

Here I will discuss the propranolol and ciprofloxacin interaction by presenting a brief case scenario. A 59 year old female with a 40-year history of smoking a pack per day presents today, complaining of worsening respiratory status. She is having a lot of dyspnea. Her COPD has responded fairly well to the long-acting anticholinergic tiotropium up until this time, so this is new to her. She has never been motivated to quit smoking and when you ask her about it, she still isn't motivated. About a week ago, she was placed on ciprofloxacin for a urinary tract infection. She has been on 4-5 different antibiotics for frequent UTI's in the last year. Since this infection started, she reports that she cannot catch her breath sometimes.

Her other diagnoses include; GERD, essential tremor, hypertension.

Medications include:
- Ranitidine
- Propranolol
- Omeprazole
- Lisinopril
- Amlodipine
- Tiotropium
- Albuterol as needed
- Ciprofloxacin

There certainly could be a lot of possibilities here that would cause worsening breathing, but if I didn't pay attention to the medications, I wouldn't be doing my job. Ciprofloxacin can inhibit CYP1A2. Propranolol is a CYP1A2 substrate. By starting ciprofloxacin in this patient, this potentially increased the concentrations of propranolol and could impact respiratory status.

Remember that beta-blockers (specifically beta-2 blockade) can cause airways to shrink. In a patient who already has difficulties breathing, this could be the difference between comfortable breathing and respiratory distress. In this scenario, you could make the argument that propranolol should be avoided altogether if possible. A frequently used alternative for essential tremor is primidone. It should be noted that this medication doesn't come without potential adverse effects and interactions as well.

The propranolol and ciprofloxacin interaction is considered a contraindication to using them together, but paying attention, educating the patient, and monitoring for adverse effects from the propranolol would be an appropriate action.

Additive Effects

Bradycardia is a major monitoring parameter for any beta-blocker. It is critical to recognize that there are numerous other medications that can cause bradycardia. When these drugs are added to a patient already taking a beta-blocker, we must pay close attention to the risk for bradycardia.

Cardiac medications like amiodarone, digoxin, and non-dihydropyridine calcium channel blockers are common agents that can contribute to a low pulse. If these medications are added or increased for a patient taking a beta-blocker, be sure to reassess the pulse following any changes. Ivabradine is a potential option used in heart failure that can also contribute to bradycardia. While typically considered as blood pressure-lowering agents, older medications like clonidine, guanfacine, and methyldopa can also contribute to bradycardia.

Drugs not used for cardiac purposes can also have the potential to cause bradycardia. Drugs that increase cholinergic activity can slow down the heart rate. Dementia medications like donepezil and rivastigmine can cause this effect. Pilocarpine and bethanechol are two other less commonly used medications that could have the cumulative effect of lowering the heart rate.

In addition to the additive effects on heart rate, blood pressure can also be affected by drugs that either raise or lower blood pressure. Drugs like stimulants can oppose the blood pressure lowering effect while other blood pressure-lowering agents like alpha-blockers have the potential to drop the blood pressure to a greater extent than we might desire.

CYP2D6 Inhibitors

Several of the commonly use beta-blockers undergo metabolic breakdown by the enzyme CYP2D6. Because of this, patients who are placed on both a CYP2D6 inhibitor and beta-blockers like metoprolol, propranolol, and carvedilol will have an increased risk of beta-blocker adverse effects. Here's a case example below.

A 71 year old male has a past medical history of hypertension. He has been on lisinopril, carvedilol, and baby aspirin. His wife has noticed that he is "down in the dumps" all the time and is wondering what is going on with him.

His primary care provider diagnoses him with depression and initiates fluoxetine. Within 2 weeks, our 71 year old male becomes dizzy and lightheaded. Blood pressure dropped along with his pulse. Undoubtedly, fluoxetine's ability to inhibit CYP2D6 likely played a role in elevating carvedilol concentrations.

What alternative action could we take to avoid this interaction? Fortunately, we have a whole list of SSRIs. Some of them can interact with CYP2D6 and others we wouldn't be quite as concerned about. In this situation, changing fluoxetine to sertraline would be a potential option. Sertraline would not have as great of a risk when it comes to inhibiting CYP2D6 and likely wouldn't impact concentrations of the carvedilol. Another alternative would be to reassess the beta-blocker being utilized. This is less desirable in this situation as the patient has been on the carvedilol without problems prior to the fluoxetine. In any event, atenolol would be a potential option that would avoid the CYP2D6 metabolic pathway and would not interact with fluoxetine. If vital signs were acceptable, a dose reduction of the carvedilol would be one other strategy to mitigate the risk of the carvedilol fluoxetine drug interaction.

Insulin and Hypoglycemia

One additional item of concern with beta-blockers is that they can blunt the signs and symptoms of hypoglycemia. While this isn't technically a true drug interaction, it is something you need to be aware of. You need to recognize that patients who are at risk for hypoglycemia may have some of the signs and symptoms of hypoglycemia blunted by beta-blockers. When I'm assessing patients' medication lists, I look to review if patients are on beta-blockers and insulin or commonly used sulfonylureas which stimulate the production and release of insulin. Patients taking insulin or sulfonylureas are at higher risk for hypoglycemia and should (at a minimum) be made aware that a beta-blocker may blunt the symptoms of hypoglycemia. This can be particularly troublesome in our geriatric patient population or those who may have impaired cognition concerns.

Thiazide Diuretics

Thiazides and Gout Treatment

A patient was being treated for hypertension, with significantly elevated systolic blood pressure. Systolic blood pressures (BP) were running in the 150-160 range. Hydrochlorothiazide was the drug that was chosen to help treat the elevated BP. The dosing was 25 mg daily. After a couple of weeks, the blood pressures were lower by about 10-15 points, and follow up kidney labs and electrolytes were stable. About a month later, this patient had an acute gout flare and a uric acid level was checked and elevated. Allopurinol was added to treat the elevation in uric acid. What was missed, however, was that hydrochlorothiazide can have the adverse effect of causing uric acid levels to increase.

While elevations in uric acid would be considered an adverse effect, this can lead to an opposition of the beneficial effects of any medication used to manage gout.

Cumulative Renal Risks

In this case scenario, we assess the importance of numerous medications potentially contributing to a case of renal failure. The higher dose thiazide diuretic is one of the medications that is likely to contribute to this concern.

A 71 year old female has a past medical history of osteoarthritis, GERD, osteoporosis, hypertension, anxiety, and depression. Her osteoarthritis has been a chronic problem and she complains of pain all over, but mainly in her hips and knees. She currently takes an occasional acetaminophen for pain.

Her current medications include:
- Omeprazole 20 mg daily
- Ranitidine 150 mg at bedtime
- Alendronate 70 mg weekly
- Calcium 500 mg BID
- Vitamin D 1,000 units daily
- Ativan 0.5 mg TID prn
- Buspirone 5 mg BID
- Zoloft 100 mg daily
- Losartan 100 mg daily
- Hydrochlorothiazide 50 mg daily

Celecoxib 200 mg BID was initiated at her last appointment by her physician. Her creatinine has now risen from 0.9 to 1.9. While celecoxib is considered better as far as reducing GI risk compared to traditional NSAIDs, it can definitely impact kidney function in a similar fashion.

What also put this patient at risk was her other medications. The hydrochlorothiazide at a relatively high dose of 50 mg daily as well as the losartan (especially in the presence of COX-2 inhibitors or NSAIDs) both can increase the risk of worsening kidney function.

Alternative medications for osteoarthritis might include trying to maximize the acetaminophen. Topical NSAIDs would be a little more challenging to justify as an alternative given that the patient reports the pain as being "all over" her body. Tramadol would be a consideration as well. Serotonin risk with tramadol isn't a huge consideration with the patient only being on sertraline 100 mg, but taking it cautiously with a small starting dose would be important. Non-pharmacologic therapies are always an important consideration and should not be overlooked.

Opposition of Beneficial Effects

This 76 year old patient was on a laundry list of blood pressure medications. Hydrochlorothiazide, losartan, metoprolol, terazosin, amlodipine, and recently had clonidine added to their regimen with minimal success. Systolic BP's still consistently ran around 160 even with aggressive treatment.

About a year ago, the patient was having really problematic pain associated with osteoarthritis and was self-treating with over-the-counter Ibuprofen 600 mg (3 of the 200 mg tabs) three times daily. The patient had never tried Tylenol(acetaminophen) in the past. Many of the increases in blood pressure medications had come in the previous year.

In addition to the use of NSAIDs, this patient has also had chronic problems with allergies. She consistently uses pseudoephedrine to help manage her symptoms. While thiazides and other antihypertensive therapy can help to effectively lower blood pressure, we must make sure that we try to avoid medications that oppose those beneficial effects. In this case, both the pseudoephedrine and the NSAID can contribute/worsen high blood pressure. Considering alternatives for both of these medications would be appropriate to help manage the risk for resistant hypertension.

Reducing the dose or the frequency of use of the pseudoephedrine would be one option. Trying to discontinue it altogether might be another potential option depending upon the severity of the symptoms and the control of her allergies. Ensuring that nasal steroids and/or newer generation antihistamine have been tried or are being used would be important to help avoid the use of the pseudoephedrine.

Thiazides and Lithium

A 42 year old male has a long history of bipolar disorder and has been well maintained on lithium. At his clinic visit today, he is having elevated blood pressure. His primary care provider initiates chlorthalidone.

Within a couple of weeks of starting the chlorthalidone, the patient shows up to an urgent care complaining of diarrhea, nausea, vomiting, fatigue, and has a modest tremor. The urgent care provider manages to recognize the drug interaction and checks a lithium level. His baseline lithium level was 0.8 which was well in the normal range. Following the interaction, the level jumped to 1.8 mEq/L. Chlorthalidone, like all thiazide diuretics, has the potential to block the excretion of lithium from the kidney. This can lead to toxicity. There are plenty of options to avoid or minimize the risk of this drug interaction. The ideal practice would be to avoid the use of chlorthalidone or any other thiazide in favor of another medication for hypertension. I must remind you to be cautious about the use of an ACE Inhibitor or ARB. These two medication classes can also interact with lithium and increase the risk of toxicity.

The alternative, if a thiazide diuretic is absolutely necessary, would be to reduce the dose of lithium. This isn't as desirable as it is always difficult to perfectly predict how much a level is going to be altered on an individual basis. A 50% reduction has been referenced in the literature, but again, it is difficult to predict exactly how much that level is going to be affected. You would also want to review how low or high the lithium level is prior to starting the medication. If it was borderline high, but still being tolerated, you'd probably be extra careful. If it was borderline low, or subtherapeutic, you might not have quite as much concern.

Cumulative Hypokalemia

Thiazide diuretics promote the loss of fluid through the urine. This loss of water also takes potassium with it. You need to be really careful when we are using thiazide diuretics in combination with loop diuretics. The situation where I've seen this combination used together is in the setting of heart failure where the patient isn't responding well enough to a loop diuretic alone. The thiazide that is most frequently used in this situation is metolazone.

Loop diuretics like furosemide are notorious for causing hypokalemia. When you add metolazone to a loop diuretic, you can get a very robust diuretic effect that can quickly lead to profound hypokalemia. This drug interaction can be fairly easily managed. The most important thing you can do is monitor electrolytes and kidney function. This will allow you to track the potassium to ensure that this interaction and the cumulative effect isn't dropping the potassium dangerously low. In the event of significant hypokalemia, supplementation can easily be added to the patient's regimen. An alternative is to reduce or stop the diuretics, but this typically isn't going to be done if kidney function remains stable and the patient still needs the diuretics for fluid loss.

I would also recommend being cautious with the use of as needed diuretic orders. Having seen a couple of patients who have been on as needed metolazone for weight gain in heart failure, you must make sure the patient understands what can happen if they take that diuretic on a consistent basis.

In one scenario, a patient was on a twice daily loop diuretic and had metolazone 2.5 mg daily PRN for weights greater than 250 lbs. This patient had a period of time where they were above 250 lbs. and began taking the metolazone regularly. They were not educated to let their provider know about the frequent use of the metolazone and how important it would be to come get labs done. They ended up getting hospitalized for profound hypokalemia. with a potassium level of 2.4 mEq/L.

Hypercalcemia Cumulative Effects

There are definitely a few medications out there that can contribute to drug-induced hypercalcemia. Here's a case scenario where the cumulative effects of calcium supplementation and thiazide diuretics led to hypercalcemia.

A 79 year old female at a long term care facility was having difficulty with hypercalcemia. Multiple different medical issues were ruled out including potential parathyroid problems as well as malignancy. Without a medical explanation, the medication regimen was reviewed for potential causes.

Upon investigation and questioning of the family, it was identified that the family was sneaking in medications to this resident without knowledge of the staff. The resident had a bottle of Tums (calcium carbonate) that she had been using "multiple" times per day for symptoms of reflux. This was obviously the first place to start and the most likely cause. The Tums was discontinued and appropriate antacid therapy was begun. Following discontinuation of the Tums, a calcium level was checked but still remained significantly elevated.

A second possible cause of the drug-induced hypercalcemia was identified. This resident was on hydrochlorothiazide for hypertension. Uniquely to thiazide diuretics (versus loops), they can actually contribute to hypercalcemia. Hydrochlorothiazide was discontinued and changed to a calcium channel blocker which resulted in the resolution of the lab abnormality.

It is important to be aware of the cumulative drug interaction risk of hypercalcemia when using calcium supplements in combination with thiazides. In addition, I'd also be aware of patients who may be taking larger doses of vitamin D. Vitamin D can also increase the cumulative risk for hypercalcemia.

Diabetes Medications and Thiazides

Thiazide diuretics have the potential to counteract the benefits of diabetes medications. The clinical significance of this interaction is dose-dependent.

This basically means that the higher the dose of the thiazide diuretic that you use, the more likely you worsen hyperglycemia in our patients with diabetes. On a scale of 1-10 for clinical significance, I'd rate this drug interaction at about a 2 or 3. With that said, if you have the option of another good blood pressure-lowering medication, you'd ideally like to avoid the thiazides.

Once a thiazide is started in a patient with diabetes, we should be able to tell how significantly the blood sugars are being elevated by monitoring blood sugars and the A1C over time. If you recognize that doses of antidiabetic agents are being increased or insulin is having to be increased, be aware if a thiazide diuretic has been started and consider reassessing if that is really needed or if alternative antihypertensive therapy would exist.

Loop Diuretics

Electrolyte Abnormalities – Cumulative Effect

Loop diuretics are very potent drugs that can run off a lot of fluid out through the kidneys. With that promotion of fluid loss, electrolytes are going to be eliminated as well. Because of this, we need to closely monitor electrolytes when initiating and changing doses. This is especially important if there are opportunities for other drugs on board to add to this effect.

Hypokalemia is one of the most important adverse effects to monitor for with loop diuretics. If left unchecked and unmonitored, they can significantly lower concentrations of potassium in the blood to a point where life-threatening cardiac changes can occur. Be sure to recognize other diuretics (i.e. thiazides) that can compound this effect.

Hyponatremia is a possibility with loop diuretics and becomes even more important to monitor for when a patient is taking a drug like desmopressin. Desmopressin on its own can cause significant hyponatremia, but when combined with another agent like a loop diuretic, it has the potential to produce profound hyponatremia.

Renal Risks

Much like all of the other diuretics, be aware of cumulative renal risks and a rising creatinine and falling GFR. Other common agents that would put a patient at greater risk of renal failure include NSAIDs, other diuretics, ACE Inhibitors or ARBs. The newer SGLT-2 agents can also have a diuretic effect that may lead to a reduction in intravascular volume and increase the risk of dehydration.

Absorption Interaction

Under normal circumstances, the oral bioavailability of furosemide is approximately 50%. Further reduction in this bioavailability can lead to an inadequate diuretic response. Cholestyramine is a medication that can bind tons of different medications in the gut and ultimately lower the systemic absorption. Be cautious with cholestyramine in the case of using loop diuretics as well as many other agents. We have so many other agents that we can use for cholesterol, so it would be best to avoid it for that indication. It is occasionally used off-label to help manage patients with frequent diarrhea. If cholestyramine can't be eliminated from the patient's medications regimen, separating the timing of administration with drugs (like furosemide) that are sensitive to the binding interaction would be essential. In the case of furosemide, if you administer furosemide 1-2 hours before the cholestyramine or 4-6 hours after the dose of cholestyramine, you should substantially minimize the risk of this binding interaction. Where this can get really tricky is when the cholestyramine or the furosemide needs to be dosed multiple times per day. Along with cholestyramine, sucralfate is another medication that is notorious for these binding interactions that lead to reduced absorption.

Methotrexate and Loop Diuretic Interaction

Methotrexate is commonly used in the setting of autoimmune diseases but also can be utilized in oncology. Loop diuretics have the potential to increase the concentrations and lead to methotrexate toxicity. If you are going to start a patient on a loop diuretic and they are on methotrexate, be sure to be aware of signs of methotrexate toxicity. Elevations in hepatic enzymes, mucositis, stomatitis, GI upset, and myelosuppression are all potential dose-dependent risks with elevated methotrexate concentrations. Educating our patients about this interaction and what signs and symptoms of toxicity to look out for would also be essential in monitoring this drug interaction.

Blood Pressure Alterations

Loop diuretics will lower blood pressure. Be aware of drugs that may increase blood pressure and agents that may contribute to a cumulative blood pressure-lowering effect. This is simply managed by monitoring blood pressure and adjusting medications accordingly.

Sulfa Allergy Interaction

Loop diuretics, with the exception of ethacrynic acid, have a sulfa group contained with the clinical structure. This can lead to numerous drug/allergy interaction flags that need to be navigated.

If a patient had a severe, life-threatening reaction to a medication with a similar sulfa group to the loop diuretics, you'd definitely want to proceed cautiously at a minimum. The first place to start in a patient with an allergy to sulfa drugs is to figure out exactly what the reaction was and which drug that reaction was from. In general, cross-reactivity between sulfa antibiotics and sulfa nonantibiotics is not common, but in the setting of a severe, life-threatening reaction, it should at least be assessed and a risk/benefit determination should be made. If the reaction was simply an intolerance, this would not prevent you from using a loop diuretic. Other nonantibiotic examples that have a sulfa group include some sulfonylureas, triptans, sulfasalazine, and thiazide diuretics.

Opposition of Edema Relieving Benefit

In the case scenario below, I outline the risk of using agents that promote fluid retention. Any drug that can cause edema is going to counteract the impact that we are trying to have with using a loop diuretic. Edema promoting agents include NSAIDs, pioglitazone, pregabalin, and gabapentin. Here's a case example:

A 68 year old male battling some knee pain tries ibuprofen 400 mg three times daily to help with osteoarthritis and muscle pain. This gentleman has a history of cardiac issues including congestive heart failure and recent heart attack. He is currently on a low dose of Lasix (furosemide) 20 mg daily for his heart failure and history of edema as well. He had talked to a neighbor who stated that he uses 800 mg three times daily – so following his neighbor's suggestion, he increases his dose to what his neighbor was taking. Within a couple of weeks, his symptoms of edema and CHF have been dramatically worsening requiring an increase in Lasix.

Upon questioning, he forgets to tell his provider that he is taking the Ibuprofen which can cause side effects like edema. This is another classic example of the prescribing cascade where a new medication causes the addition or increase of another. NSAIDs like Ibuprofen can certainly worsen CHF, oppose the diuretic effect of furosemide and cause edema as one of its side effects.

Another critical aspect of this case is patient education and appropriate assessment of all potential medications! Patients often forget, overlook, or don't recognize the fact that over the counter or herbal medications can cause problems just like prescription medications.

One last point about assessing over the counter medication and herbal medications. When they are well tolerated and used appropriately, not knowing that patients are taking them can often mask other problems or potential side effects from their prescription medications.

Spironolactone

Hyperkalemia

Spironolactone should not be used in combination with any other potassium-sparing diuretic. In addition to spironolactone, triamterene and amiloride are the two most common potassium-sparing diuretics that should be avoided in combination with spironolactone. The primary risk is hyperkalemia. Caution should also be utilized with other medications that can cause hyperkalemia.

Interestingly, in the setting of heart failure, using ACE inhibitors (or ARBs) with spironolactone can be appropriate. Spironolactone has evidence that it can improve mortality in certain types of heart failure. However, we need to closely monitor potassium levels to ensure that they are not becoming elevated. What helps us prevent hyperkalemia is that these patients are often balanced out by the use of loop diuretics which can bring down that potassium level and oppose the hyperkalemic effects of spironolactone and ACE Inhibitors.

Here's a case scenario on paying attention to potassium levels with the use of spironolactone.

My patient was having difficulty with edema and increasing the loop diuretic was not providing much additional benefit. Spironolactone was added to try to augment the fluid loss and improve CHF symptoms. This patient was already taking an ACE inhibitor and had a potassium level of around 4.8 mEq/L prior to the addition of the spironolactone. For most labs, the upper end of normal for potassium levels is about 5 mEq/L. A couple of weeks after initiation of the spironolactone, follow up electrolytes and kidney function labs were drawn and the potassium level was around 5.9 mEq/L necessitating the discontinuation of spironolactone. The bottom line, spironolactone can increase potassium levels and it is really important to have an assessment of the baseline level prior to initiating the drug. The ACE inhibitor likely contributed to hyperkalemia as well.

Renal Impairment Risk

Similar to all diuretics, spironolactone can promote the loss of fluid and deplete intravascular volume. In combination with other drugs that impair renal function, our patients may run the risk of acute renal failure.

Blood Pressure Risk

Spironolactone is commonly used in the setting of refractory hypertension. You need to be aware of medications that can both raise or lower blood pressure. Pay particular attention to those patients who require spironolactone for refractory hypertension to ensure that they are not taking agents that are raising the blood pressure and opposing the antihypertensive effect of spironolactone and/or other blood pressure reducing medications.

Triamterene

Hyperkalemia

Triamterene is primarily used in the management of hypertension. It is nearly always used in combination with hydrochlorothiazide. Triamterene is classified as a potassium-sparing diuretic. Because of this mechanism of action, you should recognize that any medication

44

that can raise potassium levels would likely have a greater risk of inducing hyperkalemia if a patient is taking triamterene.

Common examples of agents where you may have an increased risk of hyperkalemia include ACE inhibitors, ARBs, and of course, potassium supplements. Triamterene, in general, should not be utilized with other potassium sparing diuretics like spironolactone. There may be some other less common examples of medications that you haven't thought above that can contribute to hyperkalemia. Cyclosporine and heparin type products are two medications that may increase the risk of hyperkalemia. Typically heparin products are only used for shorter timeframes so the risk might not be quite as concerning but is at least something to be aware of.

Blood Pressure Risk

With triamterene, like other blood pressure lowering agents, we should be aware of medications that may have additive blood pressure lowering effects. In addition, you'll want to recognize agents that can oppose the beneficial effects of triamterene by causing hypertension.

Renal Impairment Risk

Any drug that has a diuretic effect has the potential to contribute to dehydration risks. At low doses, triamterene may not be as potent as loop diuretics. However, triamterene is no different from those other diuretics in that it could cause a cumulative type of risk if other agents that cause diuresis are on board. When a patient becomes dehydrated, this can put a strain on the kidney and if severe enough can lead to acute renal failure. Like other diuretics, be aware of agents that can cause additive insults to the kidney. Some common examples include NSAIDs, loop diuretics, thiazide diuretics, ACE inhibitors, and ARBs.

Clonidine

Cumulative Risk – CNS Depressants

Clonidine is an older medication that is on the Beers list. It is well known to cause sedation, confusion, and other CNS adverse effects. It is really important to recognize other medications that a patient may be taking to add to this cumulative side effect potential. Classic examples of drugs that are CNS depressants include benzodiazepines, skeletal muscle relaxants, opioids, and Z-drugs like zolpidem. Asking patients about sedation and confusion adverse effects, adding and increasing medications with effects slowly, and attempting to reduce these medications over time are a few strategies to try to manage this risk.

This is also a good time to mention the risk of clonidine and other CNS depressants interacting with alcohol. Patients are notorious for not disclosing that they are drinking alcohol or how much they are truly drinking. In patients (or family members) that are reporting sedation, confusion and other CNS changes, recognizing that alcohol can interact with many medications and cause a cumulative type effect is so important.

In addition to the risk of alcohol, you must inquire about the use of recreational or non-traditional drug therapies. Medical marijuana growth has been tremendous, but it comes with risks when using it in combination with other prescription medications that may have additive CNS depressant effects.

Cumulative Risk – Other Adverse Effects

SK is an 80 year old male with a history of BPH, hypertension, CAD, diabetes, and atrial fibrillation. His current medications include:

- Warfarin – goal INR 2-3
- Aspirin 81 mg daily
- Lisinopril 10 mg once daily
- Tamsulosin 0.8 mg once daily
- Finasteride 5 mg once daily
- Ibuprofen 400 mg TID PRN
- Clonidine 0.1 mg twice daily
- Unisom at bedtime

His primary concern is that he feels dizzy all the time. It is reported as being a little worse when he gets up out of his chair. He does also feel weak and faint at times. Finally, he also complains of some dry mouth.

As part of his workup, his medications need to be reviewed. With the dizziness, blood pressure would be the first assessment I would make. From there, doses of the clonidine, tamsulosin, and lisinopril all have to be reviewed. All of these medications can have orthostatic hypotension type adverse effects. Clonidine is not a very geriatric friendly medication, so this would probably be the first one I would look at getting rid of if we do have a hypotensive concern.

I would also want to assess for anemia given the use of warfarin, aspirin, and ibuprofen and also the potential physical symptoms of anemia in weakness and dizziness.

With the dry mouth reported, Unisom, which has anticholinergic activity would be a probable culprit. In addition, the clonidine can also contribute to this adverse effect. Finding non-drug interventions that might be helpful for sleep would be an excellent strategy to try to reduce the Unisom and the number of medications that can contribute to dry mouth. That is of course if the patient could be convinced of this.

Blood Pressure Effects

Like the other blood pressure-lowering agents, be aware of medications that can oppose clonidine's blood pressure-lowering effect and medications that may add to the risk of dropping blood pressure too low.

Hydralazine

Opposition of Lupus Medication

Hydroxychloroquine is a good example of an agent that can be utilized in the management of Lupus. It is important to remember that hydralazine is associated with causing a Lupus type reaction or exacerbation. In theory, hydralazine could oppose the beneficial effects that a patient with Lupus is gaining from their medications. Common medications that may be used in the management of Lupus include hydroxychloroquine, azathioprine, or methotrexate. This would be a good reason to try to avoid the use of hydralazine in favor of other antihypertensive therapy.

Blood Pressure Effects

Hydralazine is a blood pressure lowering-medication that is generally used when other agents aren't providing enough benefit or have been intolerable. This medication doesn't have a ton of unique drug interactions compared to other blood pressure agents. One of the primary reasons that it isn't used terribly often is that it does require frequent dosing which can stifle patient adherence.

Opposition or exaggeration of the blood pressure-lowering effect is the primary concern when it comes to drug interactions. Be aware of agents added to hydralazine that may alter the blood pressure and monitor accordingly.

Are you finding this book helpful? I'd love a kind review on Amazon if you have a chance! If you have feedback on improvement or notice something isn't quite right, feel free to shoot me an email at: mededucation101@gmail.com

CYP3A4 Inhibition

Statins are frequently used medications for cardiovascular prevention. Atorvastatin and rosuvastatin are the two most commonly used statins. One important fact to remember is that atorvastatin will tend to be a little more impacted by CYP3A4 inhibition compared to rosuvastatin. It is important to remember this in the event that you are trying to determine which one you'd like to use as both can be classified as high-intensity statins that are necessary for our higher risk cardiovascular patients.

The big challenge with CYP3A4 inhibitors is that there are a LOT of them. Immunosuppressants like cyclosporine, antibiotics like clarithromycin, antifungals like fluconazole, gout medications like colchicine, blood pressure medications like most of the calcium channel blockers, and even many HIV medications can all inhibit CYP3A4 and increase the risk of elevating statin concentrations.

For some patients, atorvastatin is a little bit cheaper than rosuvastatin so that is a consideration, but if you know you are likely to run into some of these drug interactions over time, it would be ideal to try to minimize the risk of CYP3A4 interactions by utilizing rosuvastatin.

CYP3A4 Inducers

On the flipside of the spectrum, recognizing CYP3A4 inducers for patients taking many of the statins is important. CYP3A4 inducers will do the exact opposite in that they will reduce the concentrations of statins. In a patient at higher cardiovascular risk, this is a big concern as they will not be as adequately protected from a future cardiovascular event as they should be.

Classic examples of drugs that will induce CYP3A4 include carbamazepine, phenytoin, phenobarbital, primidone, and rifampin. Identifying these agents when statins are on board is important to recognize why a patient may not be responding to statin therapy. We can assess this by looking at lipid levels over time.

Rosuvastatin avoids the CYP3A4 pathway. In the event you are having to deal with atorvastatin or simvastatin interacting with some of these inducers, rosuvastatin will be a potential option to help avoid the risk of therapeutic failure.

Statins and Red Yeast Rice

I often get referrals for patients who have questions about supplements. Some will ask me "Should I take all these supplements?" There are definitely some scenarios where I think supplements may be a good option and worth taking, but often times I think patients are just wasting their money. Here's a scenario of a patient taking red yeast rice and the risk that is associated in combination with a statin.

A 63 year old male has a PMH of BPH, OA, GERD, Atopic dermatitis, diabetes, and hypertension. His current medication list including supplements includes:
- Atorvastatin 40 mg daily
- Metformin 500 mg BID
- Cinnamon 1,000 mg once daily
- Glucosamine/chondroitin 500 mg TID
- Vitamin E 400 units per day
- Multivitamin once daily
- Vitamin C 500 mg daily
- Ferrous sulfate 325 mg daily
- Lisinopril 10 mg daily
- B12 500 mg daily
- Red yeast rice 200 mg daily
- Omeprazole 20 mg daily

There is some evidence that red yeast rice has a statin component in it. The really difficult thing with supplements is that they are not well studied. Exactly how much cholesterol-lowering effect red yeast rice and how well it reduces the risk of cardiovascular outcomes isn't well known. When comparing red yeast rice to statins as far as reducing the risk of MI and other issues, the statin is obviously going to have a lot better research behind it. I would recommend discontinuing the red yeast rice and continuing the statin.

There is the risk from this drug interaction that we are doubling up on the statin and that could potentially precipitate as statin toxicity. Most concerning would be the risk of rhabdomyolysis.

Statins and Grapefruit Juice

Patients often don't understand drug interactions. In this scenario, I'll discuss the statin and grapefruit juice interaction and really what we can do about it. Upon assessment of a patient's medications, your patient reports that she isn't taking her statin medication. She has a past history of heart attack, stroke, as well as type 2 diabetes. She is certainly at risk of future cardiac and stroke events and the use of a statin is a must if possible.

When questioned why she wasn't taking her simvastatin, she had stated that she was taking grapefruit juice and that she believed that the grapefruit juice would do the same thing. The statin and grapefruit juice interaction doesn't quite work that way. In the patient's defense, it was never explained to her how the interaction works. After explaining this, she understood that the grapefruit juice likely wasn't benefitting her as far as reducing her risk of heart attack and stroke.

Grapefruit juice is a potent inhibitor of the CYP3A4 enzyme which is responsible for the breakdown of many of the statins. Atorvastatin, simvastatin, and lovastatin will be affected the most by this drug interaction as these statins are metabolized by CYP3A4. Rosuvastatin and pravastatin will be less impacted by this drug interaction.

She still stated she was going to do her grapefruit or grapefruit juice every morning because it really makes her feel good. In this situation, it makes the most sense to switch simvastatin to pravastatin or maybe more likely since she is at such high risk for future problems, a higher intensity statin like rosuvastatin which will likely not have the same interaction as the simvastatin would. Another potential option would be to continue the simvastatin and monitor labs and looking out for signs and symptoms of statin toxicity. I probably prefer a switch since she wasn't taking the medication anyway at this point in time.

Gemfibrozil and Statins

Gemfibrozil and statins present an interesting drug interaction that needs to be addressed. How should we address the interaction?

The first question to ask is, do other alternatives exist? Other alternatives to the statin are probably unlikely as many patients have cardiovascular disease or other clinical concerns that necessitate its use. With gemfibrozil, however, we do potentially have other options like fenofibrate or niacin which may interact with the statins to a lesser extent.

Clinically, we also need to assess the severity of the situation. In addition, we should be aware of what indication the gemfibrozil is being used for. Gemfibrozil will almost exclusive be used for elevated triglycerides. Elevated triglycerides can raise the risk of acute pancreatitis.

Are the triglycerides 400, or are they 1600 makes a substantial difference as to the seriousness with which they should be treated.

If all else fails, and if a provider is adamant about continuing with gemfibrozil and a statin, monitoring and education is an absolute must. The biggest risk with this interaction is rhabdomyolysis, so assessment of CPK might be an appropriate way to help monitor for the potential interaction between gemfibrozil and statins.

Depending upon labs, cardiovascular risk, and pancreatitis risk, another alternative to consider may be to reduce the dose of one and/or the other agent.

As a pharmacist, I am trained to look at agents that can cause what we are trying to treat. Antipsychotics are an example that comes to mind when I think about the possibility of drug-induced hypertriglyceridemia.

Additive Effects – Daptomycin

Daptomycin is an antibiotic that can be utilized in the treatment of non-pneumonia MRSA. The drug itself is unique in that it is one of the few drugs (besides statins) that can cause rhabdomyolysis.

With the understanding that daptomycin can cause rhabdomyolysis on its own, we should recognize that when using it with a statin, we will increase this risk further.

How should we manage this? Because daptomycin duration of therapy will likely be very short, the easiest strategy to manage this potential interaction is to hold the statin while the antibiotic for infection is given. The use of daptomycin will likely be necessary, but there is an off chance that we could give an alternative antibiotic agent that can cover MRSA or whatever other bacteria we may be treating.

Clopidogrel

CYP2C19 Interactions

Clopidogrel is a very important antiplatelet agent that can be used to help reduce the risk of heart attack and stroke. One of the complexities with clopidogrel's pharmacokinetics involves its interaction with the CYP enzyme system. Clopidogrel is a prodrug which means that the active compound ingested does not have the clinical activity. Enzymes in the body must convert it to the active compound. This activation is primarily done by CYP2C19.

Alterations in the enzyme due to drugs or genetic variation can lead to alterations in the clinical response. In the below case scenario, I discuss some of the possible reasons as to why a patient may not respond to clopidogrel.

A 62-year-old male had a heart attack about 9 months ago. He was stented and placed on both aspirin 81 mg daily and clopidogrel 75 mg daily. He presents today to the emergency department and is diagnosed with a STEMI. His wife is wondering why the medications used to prevent this from happening didn't work. Below I assess 3 possible reasons for clopidogrel failure.

Step one in any investigation about treatment failure is to assess patient adherence. When I'm dealing with a patient who is living at home and taking care of their own medications, I always put a large emphasis on adherence. This is one of the most common reasons as to why a medication doesn't work. In addition to gently approaching (avoiding accusation) this with the patient, I would also like to get the dispensing records from the pharmacy to verify that he was routinely picking this medication up.

With the growing practice of pharmacogenomics, we have to consider that this patient may have a variation of CYP2C19 that does not allow him to adequately metabolize the drug to its active form. Clopidogrel is a prodrug that requires activation by CYP2C19. This should be investigated and alternative antiplatelet therapy considered.

CYP2C19 can be affected by numerous medications. By blocking CYP2C19 action, it could result in a reduced therapeutic effect. The extent of the clinical implication of each of these drug interactions still remains debatable. However, in a patient who has had a repeat event, we must consider this possibility. I would look at the timing of new medications and dose changes. Examples of common medications that could reduce the effectiveness of clopidogrel include omeprazole, cimetidine, esomeprazole, fluoxetine, and fluconazole.

In addition to tradition prescription drug therapy, there is potential for supplements to cause this drug interaction. Grapefruit juice has been reported to reduce the effectiveness of clopidogrel. Recommending patients avoid grapefruit juice, in general, is a good idea given the number of drug interactions that can occur because of its use. If a patient is unwilling to make changes in their grapefruit juice consumption, we should ensure that they are educated about the potential risks with regards to drug interactions.

Omeprazole Clopidogrel Clinical Controversy

The omeprazole clopidogrel interaction has always been a challenging one to know precisely what to do. Since a significant number of media reports came out in 2010 due to information regarding the omeprazole and clopidogrel interaction, it has been hotly debated as to how to manage this drug interaction.

Omeprazole can reduce the serum concentrations of the active metabolite of clopidogrel. If we connect the dots, we can likely suspect that this will impact our patients clinically. At the time of putting this book together, clinical studies have never been done to show negative outcomes data. So what should we do with this interaction?

I'll propose some questions you should think about when managing this interaction.

How long has the patient been on clopidogrel? Remember that clopidogrel is often used for a limited time following stenting. Make sure to look at the indication for clopidogrel. We may be able to discontinue clopidogrel and not have to worry about the interaction.

Can aspirin be substituted? Often aspirin is going to be utilized prior to clopidogrel, but rarely you may run into a situation where a patient is on clopidogrel alone. Be sure to ask the question and investigate if the patient has tried aspirin. Keep in mind here that the indication does matter as well.

Is the PPI required long term? PPIs are some of the most highly utilized medications and often we can get by with an H2 blocker or even a trial taper off the PPI. Be sure the GI indication for the PPI is reviewed and assess if we can somehow get off the PPI.

Is a switch to a different PPI like pantoprazole appropriate? Pantoprazole has less risk of inhibiting CYP2C19 compared to omeprazole or esomeprazole. This can be a pretty simple switch, but insurance, efficacy, or tolerability challenges can exist.

Antiplatelet Activity

Because clopidogrel inhibits the activity of platelets, the most recognizable side effect is the risk of a bleed. This can be compounded by numerous medications. Aspirin, anticoagulants, and NSAIDs are a few of the most common agents that can increase the risk of bleeding.

When anticoagulants or aspirin is used in combination with clopidogrel, we must monitor these patients closely for bleeding risk. There are several ways that we can do this. Measuring hemoglobin (or hematocrit) can be helpful in trying to identify patients who have had blood loss or higher risk patients where blood loss could be life-threatening. Along with the hemoglobin, we can also periodically assess platelets to ensure that patients have adequate ability to slow down the blood loss in the event they have a laceration or some sort of tissue damage.

Educating patients about the risks of antiplatelet therapy is critical. They can help us as healthcare professionals monitor for signs and symptoms of bleeding. Encouraging them to report new issues or concerns is essential. In addition to bleeding, having patients report significant bruising or bruising that is occurring without knowledge of trauma or injury is very important to assess the safety of antiplatelet medications and those who may be on more than one medication that can increase the risk of a bleed.

What to do with antiplatelet medications in the setting of anemia has always been a huge challenge for me. Here's a scenario with some questions to think about. A 64 year old female has a history of CAD, hyperlipidemia, hypertension, CABG, depression, anemia, osteoarthritis, and constipation. Current meds include:
- Lisinopril 5 mg daily
- Clopidogrel 75 mg daily
- Crestor 20 mg daily
- Metoprolol tartrate 25 mg daily
- Sertraline 25 mg daily
- FeSO4 325 mg daily
- Colace 100 mg BID
- Diclofenac 50 mg BID

Labs:

- Hemoglobin 9.6
- Platelets 78

When assessing anemia, the first thing I would look at would be the labs. How low are the hemoglobin/hematocrit/platelets? Also, have they always been this low or is a recent drop obvious?

Patient symptoms are important. Is there blood loss (i.e. blood in the stool or recent surgery)? Are they bruising easily? Are they feeling fatigued? These are all important questions.

Before assessing the antiplatelet medication, I look at all the other medications. The most obvious one is diclofenac. I would seek an alternative here or recommend assessing for GI bleed risk if the NSAID is deemed necessary. With the patient's osteoarthritis history, acetaminophen would make some sense to inquire about. GI prophylaxis may be appropriate if the NSAID needs to stay. There is some evidence that SSRIs can impact platelet function. At the dose of sertraline 25 mg daily, I would not suspect that this is playing a large role in comparison to the NSAID and clopidogrel.

The timing of when clopidogrel and diclofenac were started would be another factor in trying to identify a medication-related cause.

It's important for us to remember that there are tons of medical reasons for thrombocytopenia and anemia. If medications are ruled out, be sure that our other healthcare providers assess for medical considerations.

Aspirin

Cumulative Bleed Risk

Aspirin is well known to increase the risk of a bleed. This potential risky adverse effect is also what gives the drug its benefit in reducing the risk of heart attack and stroke. From a drug interaction aspect, the most significant risk of bleeding can be exacerbated by other medications that can increase the risk of bleeding.

Anticoagulation, antiplatelet medications, and NSAIDs can all play a role in increasing bleed risk by inhibiting the action of platelets or clotting factors.

One question that has come up in clinical practice is the use of baby aspirin in combination with NSAIDs for pain management. This can be done in most situations, but we have to be aware that this combination is going to increase the risk of a bleed. I would also recommend avoiding some of the higher risk GI NSAIDs. Ketorolac specifically is one of the highest risk NSAIDs when it comes to its ability to cause a GI bleed. Indomethacin is another example of a higher GI risk NSAID.

Recognizing the fact that NSAIDs are available over the counter is critical. We must ask patients about over-the-counter and supplement use. There are supplements that have been associated with increased bleed risk and/or have antiplatelet activity. Garlic and Ginkgo supplements have been associated with platelet inhibition effects. In the majority of cases, there is not enough evidence for me to recommend garlic or ginkgo supplements for any specific indication. I do educate patients about this risk with supplements and the use of aspirin or any other agent that can increase the bleed risk.

The SSRIs have come up in the literature and you will see this interaction with aspirin. In theory, SSRIs may potentiate the bleed risk effect of aspirin. How clinically significant is this interaction and would we do any additional monitoring because of this? The clinical significance is debatable. At this point in time, there are no prospective, randomized controlled trials on whether the SSRIs increase the risk of bleeding, but we do have lots of retrospective data.

Bottom line, there is a definite likelihood that an SSRI inhibits the function of platelets. The extent of that inhibition and clinical impact is debatable. Clinical reasoning, monitoring, and common sense are probably the best we can do right now. Assessing CBC and educating patients to monitor for signs and symptoms of bleeding is the best advice at this point. Keep in mind, you are probably likely to do this regardless even if a patient is simply taking aspirin without an SSRI.

Aspirin and Lisinopril

I was at a long term care facility and had a patient on lisinopril 10 mg daily for hypertension as well as Aspirin 325 mg daily for cardiovascular prophylaxis. This was flagged by a drug interaction program and the pharmacy faxed a physician to address this situation. The risk of this interaction is that aspirin can blunt the antihypertensive effects of lisinopril.

Putting myself in this situation, this is a great case where a solution could be offered rather than just notifying the physician. There are two solutions that initially come to my mind.

This patient was a resident of a long term care facility. The facility should have good information on the blood pressure results of this resident. The individual who was prompted with this interaction could certainly pick up the phone and inquire nursing staff about the blood pressure readings. Monitoring is so important when it comes to drug interactions, and this option tends to slip through the cracks once in a while as I've seen some providers almost panic and not think about what the alert is actually saying.

The second solution would be to ask the provider to assess the current dose of aspirin. This interaction doesn't occur or has a minimal clinical effect when the dose of Aspirin is less than 100 mg daily. In many cases, we can get by with a dose of 81 mg daily.

CKD and CHF Risk

Aspirin is classified as an NSAID. With any NSAID, there is a risk of exacerbating or causing acute renal failure. In addition to the renal failure risk, there is a risk of exacerbating heart failure.

Very seldom do patients use aspirin as an analgesic or anti-inflammatory medication. However, if used at higher doses for this purpose, aspirin can certainly increase the risk of renal failure and/or edema which could exacerbate heart failure. When patients are taking the standard baby dose aspirin for cardiovascular prophylaxis, the concern of renal failure or CHF exacerbation is not as concerning.

If you have a patient who is taking analgesic dosages (i.e. 325-650 mg) multiple times per day, we have to worry about the potential insult to the kidney and exacerbation of heart failure. As far as the renal concerns go, I'd be looking to minimize the chance for multiple drugs that can cause renal impairment. The combination of diuretics, ACE Inhibitors or ARBs, and the use of higher-dose aspirin can substantially increase the risk for renal impairment.

When it comes to heart failure and higher doses of aspirin, these should generally be avoided. They can oppose the beneficial effects of diuretics by exacerbating edema.

Methotrexate and Aspirin Interaction

Aspirin has the potential to increase the concentrations of methotrexate. The major question with this interaction is whether the baby dose aspirin will cause clinically significant elevations in methotrexate concentrations. It seems to be a dose-dependent effect, so the likelihood of methotrexate toxicity following administration of a baby dose of aspirin is probably extremely low.

Buffered Aspirin and Binding Interactions

You have to remember that buffered aspirin is different from regular aspirin. Buffered aspirin is essentially paired with an antacid medication in the same tablet. While this can be beneficial in helping to prevent stomach upset and heartburn type symptoms, it can also cause binding interactions.

Buffered aspirin will often contain calcium or magnesium which can cause a whole host of interactions that will reduce the absorption and concentration of other medications. Of highest importance are antibiotics. Drugs from the quinolone and tetracycline class of drugs can be bound up by the "buffering agent" in buffered aspirin. This will lead to lower concentrations and potential treatment failure.

The easiest way to avoid the potential for these binding interactions is to encourage your patients who need to take a prophylactic dose of aspirin to utilize regular aspirin or the enteric-coated version of aspirin. If patients absolutely feel as if they need buffered aspirin, you can alternate the timing of the doses of the aspirin and interacting antibiotic so they are not coadministered close to one another. For example, taking levofloxacin in the evening and taking the buffered aspirin in the morning would be sufficient to avoid the risk for this binding interaction.

Warfarin

CYP2C9 Inhibition

Warfarin's metabolism is most significantly impacted by CYP2C9. Inhibition of CYP2C9 is going to lead to elevated concentrations of warfarin and an elevated INR. There are numerous examples of drugs that can inhibit CYP2C9 that you should be aware of. Amiodarone, tamoxifen, sulfamethoxazole, and fluconazole are some common examples. Metronidazole is another common example as demonstrated by this case scenario.

A 74 year old female was recently discharged from the hospital with pneumonia. The latest INR was 2.1.

Current Meds:
- Aspirin 81 mg daily

- Warfarin 2.5 mg daily
- Lamotrigine 25 mg BID
- Ranitidine 150 mg daily
- Carafate 1 gram twice daily
- Loperamide as needed (just recently started)
- Ramipril 5 mg daily
- Amlodipine 10 mg daily
- Metoprolol 100 mg twice daily

About 3 days following discharge she begins to develop foul-smelling diarrhea. It continued for another 2-3 days before going into the clinic to get assessed.

Stool testing was completed. The diagnosis was made as a C. diff infection. The patient had not been able to tolerate oral vancomycin in the past so she was initiated on metronidazole for 10 days to treat the suspected infection. On day 7 of antibiotic therapy, the patient has a nose bleed that she cannot resolve. She goes to a local urgent care clinic where an INR was checked and it was 9.4.

So, we must ask the question as to what would've prevented the warfarin and metronidazole interaction from getting out of control and putting our patient at risk? Taking warfarin and metronidazole will usually result in increased concentrations of warfarin and increase the risk of elevated INR. Checking an INR on day 3-5 would have been a plausible option and may have been able to prevent this interaction from getting out of hand.

Another option that I occasionally see in practice is preemptive dose reduction of warfarin. I've seen dose reductions in the range of 30-50%, but this is likely going to be difficult to predict and may be variable from patient to patient.

Another alternative would be to identify if the patient is a candidate for a newer oral anticoagulant that might have a lower risk of interactions in the future.

Alternative Breakdown Pathways

One of the reasons why warfarin has so many potential drug interactions is because it is broken down by several metabolic enzymes. In addition to being primarily metabolized by CYP2C9, it is in part broken down by CYP3A4, CYP1A2, and CYP2C19. The extent of this breakdown and what enzymes an interacting drug with

60

inhibit or induce will play a significant role in how clinically serious the drug interaction is. It is critical to assess INR following medication changes that may impact these metabolic pathways.

Enzyme Induction

Because warfarin is broken down by enzymatic action in the liver, many of the classic enzyme inducers can impact the blood concentrations of the drug. This can ultimately lead to the risk of treatment failure. Treatment failure can result in serious consequences like DVT, pulmonary embolism, or stroke.

Classic examples of enzyme inducers include carbamazepine, St. John's Wort, and rifampin. In the rifampin section, you can read about a case scenario where warfarin concentrations skyrocketed after rifampin was discontinued.

Cumulative Bleed Risk

Much like aspirin, clopidogrel, or any other anticoagulant, drugs that cause bleeding that are used in combination with other drugs that cause bleeding should be avoided, or at a minimum used with extreme caution.

One question that has come up several times is the risk of using triple therapy. In patients with atrial fibrillation who are at risk for stroke, they will likely be on anticoagulation. This may be warfarin, apixaban, rivaroxaban or another agent. Patients who have atrial fibrillation may also have a heart attack and need stent placement. Current guidelines recommend dual antiplatelet therapy with aspirin and a P2Y12 inhibitor like clopidogrel. Can patients be on all three of these? There is not an easy answer to this question. In some cases, patients can be on all three blood-thinning medications, and in some cases, they probably shouldn't be. There is a clinical determination that needs to be made on a case by case basis where the risk of bleed is weighed against the risk for heart attack and stroke. Keep in mind that this risk determination may change as clinical circumstances change or as a patient ages.

Warfarin and Phenytoin

This one is complicated. Warfarin is one of those medications that is highly albumin bound. A drug that is bound to proteins in the blood cannot have physiologic activity. Phenytoin is also highly protein-bound. When phenytoin is administered, it can kick warfarin off of those proteins in the blood. This can lead to more free warfarin around to do its blood-thinning thing. Higher unbound, or free drug concentrations results in more warfarin activity and higher INRs.

On the flipside, phenytoin is a notorious CYP enzyme inducer. Because of enzyme induction by phenytoin, this may reduce the concentrations of warfarin. Bottom line: it is critical to monitor INR closely in patients where these agents are used together. There is also the potential for phenytoin toxicity risk to be increased in a patient starting warfarin. My advice is to be incredibly careful with this combination and avoid it if possible. Also, be aware of dose changes for either medication as this may alter concentrations of the other drug.

Levofloxacin and Warfarin

A 69 year old female was recently diagnosed with pneumonia and placed on levofloxacin (Levaquin). She is also taking warfarin.

So what does protein, vitamin K, and drug metabolism have to do with anything?
There are 3 proposed mechanisms that the levofloxacin warfarin drug interaction occurs by.

Warfarin is bound to protein in the blood. When it is bound to protein, it cannot cause the blood-thinning effect. There is the potential that levofloxacin can "kick" warfarin off of these protein sites, leaving more warfarin freely available to go into action, thin the blood and subsequently raise the INR.

Levofloxacin kills bacteria. Some of those bacteria in the gut produce vitamin K for the body. Vitamin K opposes (and is the antidote) the action of warfarin. Less vitamin K can increase warfarin's effects and raise the INR

The last proposed mechanism for this drug interaction is that levofloxacin blocks the liver from breaking down warfarin. More warfarin in the system can lead to more blood-thinning effects and a rise in INR.

So, how concerned should we be about this interaction? When not closely or appropriately monitored, I have seen this interaction cause significant bleeding. On a scale of mild/moderate/severe, I would put it at a moderate. She should be monitored for an increased risk of bleeding. Her healthcare team will likely check an INR in 3-5 days once levofloxacin is started. If it is above the normal target, they will likely have to reduce the dose of warfarin and continue to monitor the INR closely. If the INR is elevated and the dose of warfarin is reduced, it is important to remember that when levofloxacin is discontinued, she may run the risk of having her INR go below the target range.

Amiodarone and Warfarin

JT is a 61 year old male. He has recently been diagnosed with atrial fibrillation and placed on amiodarone. He is also on warfarin with a history of DVT/PE. The amiodarone and warfarin interaction can be a little more challenging than other drug interactions. What really makes this unique is the long duration of action and half-life of amiodarone.

Important information on the pharmacokinetics of amiodarone:
- Onset: 2 days to 3 weeks
- Peak effect: 1 week to 5 months
- Half-life: average 58 days

Here are some questions to consider when identifying a patient on amiodarone and warfarin.
How long have they been on these agents? This can help you determine if an interaction remains relevant or is already accounted for in INR monitoring.

How often is it reasonable to check INR when first initiating the amiodarone? Patient factors are going to play a role in this question. Due to the unique pharmacokinetics of amiodarone, this interaction can take up to weeks to ramp up. Checking a couple of times per week or once a week would potentially be reasonable until we feel the patient has stabilized.

Is the patient a candidate for a newer oral anticoagulant that might not have this concern? One way to manage an interaction is to avoid one of the interacting medications. This isn't always possible, but should always be reviewed.

How long are we going to more closely monitor the amiodarone and warfarin interaction? If we've done weekly checks for 2, 3, 4 weeks with no change in an INR that is at goal, most clinicians will go back to routine monthly monitoring.

Vitamin K and Warfarin

When I think about drug interactions, what a patient is eating isn't the first thing that comes to mind. Warfarin is definitely an exception to this mindset. Vitamin K intake can substantially alter INR and the effectiveness or ineffectiveness of warfarin. One of the critical questions you should ask when assessing a patient's INR that is out of range is "Have you recently had any diet changes that are out of the ordinary?"

Some of the more common foods that contain significant amounts of vitamin K include green, leafy vegetables. Specific examples of high vitamin K foods include broccoli, kale, spinach, collard greens, and Brussel sprouts. Liver and lighter meats like chicken and pork may also contain some vitamin K.

With vitamin K, there is an inverse relationship with INR. As intake goes up, the INR will go down. In the same respect, if there is a substantial reduction in vitamin K intake (i.e. maybe your patient is sick and not eating well), the INR will likely go up. If you remember that the antidote to warfarin is vitamin K, this should help remember the inverse relationship.

NSAIDs

NSAIDs are notoriously associated with GI bleeding. Because of their ability to directly damage the GI tract and inhibit the activity of platelets, NSAIDs are the most common medication associated with causing GI ulcers. This risk is amplified by the use of warfarin. I discuss this interaction in more detail in the NSAID section.

Fenofibrate

Rhabdomyolysis Risk

Fenofibrate is most often utilized in the management of very high triglycerides. Triglycerides generally aren't a priority target unless they are substantially elevated or the patient has other risk factors for pancreatitis. We generally don't even consider treating triglycerides until the patient's level hit at least 500 mg/dL. Even in that situation, if a patient is at low risk for pancreatitis, we may wait until they get even higher than that.

Many patients with elevated triglycerides will also have elevations in LDL. Many may be at risk for cardiovascular disease and there may be indications for both statin therapy and fibrate therapy. If this is the case, we must remember that fenofibrate can interact with statins and increase the risk of rhabdomyolysis.

In monitoring this drug interaction, the first thing I review is if both a statin and fibrate are necessary. If they are, educating patients about signs and symptoms of myopathy and rhabdomyolysis should be a part of their care plan. We also monitor for risk if patients are displaying symptoms or are concerned about this interaction due to past history of clinical concerns. Checking a CPK can help assess for drug-induced rhabdomyolysis if the patient is reporting symptoms consistent with that diagnosis.

It is important to note that fenofibrate is likely to carry a lower risk of rhabdomyolysis compared to the use of gemfibrozil. If you have a patient who absolutely needs triglyceride-lowering therapy and the debate is between fenofibrate and gemfibrozil, fenofibrate will likely be your preferred choice when considering the safety aspect of these agents in combination with statins.

Fenofibrate and Cyclosporine

When we have patients who are taking immunosuppressive agents for a transplant, we have to be extremely careful with drug interactions. These patients will typically have a transplant team that helps with medication management. However, it is critical to recognize that many of the drugs used in transplantation can have drug interactions.

Fenofibrate has the potential to lower the concentrations of cyclosporine. The amount that concentrations will be reduced will be variable from patient to patient. Our best strategy would be to avoid using fenofibrate unless there is a strong indication to use it. In the event that it would be necessary to use fenofibrate, we would absolutely have to communicate with the patient's transplant team and ensure that levels were being monitored.

Fenofibrate and Warfarin

Fenofibrate has the potential to raise warfarin concentrations. This drug interaction is suspected to happen via mild CYP2C9 inhibition. Fenofibrate isn't likely to inhibit CYP2C9 to the extent of metronidazole or sulfamethoxazole, but with the narrow therapeutic index window of warfarin, this is still something we are going to have to monitor. Educating the patient about bleed risks and checking INR following initiation of fenofibrate would be the most essential tasks of management.

Rivaroxaban

CYP3A4 and P-glycoprotein Inducers

There are a few drugs that are considered strong inducers of CYP3A4 and P-glycoprotein. These drugs essentially speed up the metabolic activity of CYP3A4 and can break down drugs that use this pathway for elimination more quickly. Increasing the activity of P-glycoprotein will also likely contribute to lower concentrations of rivaroxaban. Some of the more common examples include carbamazepine, Fosphenytoin, phenytoin, phenobarbital, primidone, St. John's wort, and rifampin. Looking for alternatives to these agents, or switching to a different anticoagulant will likely be essential.

The major risk with using these inducers with rivaroxaban is treatment failure. Treatment failure can be catastrophic when using a high risk/high reward anticoagulant. Unlike warfarin, we do not base the dosing of drug on INR so there is no way to safely increase the dose of rivaroxaban to overcome this enzyme induction risk. If we did increase the dose, we don't have evidence to lean on to accurately say how much higher we would need to go.

St. John's Wort is a supplement that can also induce CYP3A4 and P-glycoprotein. I cannot recall a situation where I would ever recommend a patient should take St. John's Wort. The risk of drug interactions both present and future is too great for patients to take this supplement.

CYP3A4 and P-glycoprotein Inhibitors

Because rivaroxaban's metabolism does depend on CYP3A4, there is significant potential for drug interactions. In general, the more potent the effects on CYP3A4, the more concerned you should be. By inhibiting CYP3A4 (and P-glycoprotein), we run the opposite risk of induction. The inhibition of both of these will likely lead to the risk of supratherapeutic levels and increase the opportunity for bleeding.

This is definitely a bit of a gray area in attempting to decide whether to monitor for increased bleed risk or absolutely avoid these agents altogether. Avoidance of drugs like ketoconazole, itraconazole, and ritonavir is recommended. Examples of agents with stronger inhibition

66

of CYP3A4 and P-glycoprotein that may be considered to continue together but monitor include erythromycin, clarithromycin, and verapamil. The ideal advice is to find alternatives to all of these agents so we don't increase the bleed risk for our patients.

Cobicistat is a medication used as a pharmacokinetic booster in HIV therapy. This is a contraindicated medication with rivaroxaban that has the potential to raise concentrations of rivaroxaban. It can potently inhibit CYP3A4.

Opposing Effects

Rivaroxaban can be a lifesaving drug by preventing blood clots. It is critical to recognize medications that may raise the risk of a blood clot and directly oppose the beneficial effects of rivaroxaban or any other anticoagulant. Estrogen therapy is commonly used in postmenopausal women for menopausal symptoms and for birth control in premenopausal women. It has the potential to cause blood clots and in patients who need anticoagulation to prevent blood clots, estrogen should be avoided.

Rivaroxaban Bleed Risk

Rivaroxaban is an anticoagulant that is most commonly used to prevent stroke or manage a DVT/PE. It ultimately thins the blood. It should never be used in combination with another anticoagulant like warfarin, apixaban, dabigatran, etc. As discussed in the clopidogrel and aspirin section, when we have multiple agents on board that have similar effects of increasing bleed risk, that patient is at a much higher risk of bleeding than if they were only on one agent. Patient monitoring, lab monitoring, and the continual need for a risk versus benefit analysis is absolutely necessary.

While rivaroxaban is contraindicated with other oral anticoagulants, there may be situations where aspirin and/or clopidogrel may be used in combination with rivaroxaban. There may be one extremely rare situation where you may be on both rivaroxaban and warfarin for a few days. Because warfarin takes a while to get to therapeutic INR levels, a patient may continue to require anticoagulation while that warfarin gets to therapeutic levels. In the conversion of rivaroxaban to warfarin, you may continue to give the rivaroxaban for a few days in combination with the warfarin until the warfarin gets to its desired therapeutic level.

Much like with warfarin and other anticoagulants, we should try to avoid the use of NSAIDs. The GI bleed risk is substantially raised with this combination. In some situations, there may not be ideal alternatives for pain management. In that situation, GI protection with an H2 blocker or PPI should be considered. In addition, minimizing the dose and monitoring increased bleed risk through checking a periodic CBC would be critical. Patient education about potential risks and what they can monitor for would also be essential.

Apixaban

CYP3A4 and P-glycoprotein Inducers

When the NOACs (sometimes referred to as DOACs) first came out they were heavily promoted as having fewer drug interactions compared to warfarin. This is true, but please remember that "fewer drug interactions" doesn't mean "no drug interactions".

Much like with rivaroxaban, drugs that induce CYP3A4 and P-glycoprotein can lower concentrations of apixaban to dangerous levels and precipitate treatment failure. Medications that can have this effect that I've seen used in clinical practice include carbamazepine, phenytoin, primidone, rifampin, and phenobarbital. Below I discuss a case scenario regarding apixaban and carbamazepine and strategies for managing this interaction.

A 72-year-old has a past medical history of atrial fibrillation, hypertension, hypercholesterolemia, osteoarthritis, and painful trigeminal neuralgia. He was recently transitioned off of warfarin to apixaban. The primary reason for this was he was tired of having to do INRs every month. A secondary reason was the new guideline recommendations regarding preference for NOACs in atrial fibrillation.

The major drug interaction with his medications was the carbamazepine apixaban interaction. Carbamazepine is a strong enzyme inducer and can substantially lower concentrations of apixaban. The same thing can also happen with warfarin, but we can adjust by monitoring INR.

With this drug interaction, it is recommended to avoid using these medications together. If this is the goal, then your objective is simple. You must change either the carbamazepine or the apixaban to avoid the drug interaction.

In this patient scenario, carbamazepine is being used for the indication of trigeminal neuralgia. Trying to wean off this medication to avoid the carbamazepine apixaban interaction would probably be the ideal strategy.

This is totally dependent upon the effectiveness of the drug and the patient's desire to continue with it. It is essential to consider the patient's goals, past history, and desires in doing any sort of transition or discontinuation.

While carbamazepine has the best evidence in the setting of trigeminal neuralgia, other options might be considered. Gabapentin and baclofen are two agents that I have seen used in the past.

If the carbamazepine has had life-altering benefit and the patient will not go without it, we would be between a rock and a hard place. However, if the only reason that the patient wanted to switch to the apixaban was due to less lab monitoring, they might continue to accept the inconvenience of routine INRs to continue with the carbamazepine.

What about leaving it and adjusting doses? The problem with this strategy is that we aren't really sure how much apixaban concentrations are going to be affected by the interaction. This could vary greatly due to a whole host of factors like dosing, genetics, adherence, etc. So while we know that concentrations of apixaban will likely be subtherapeutic with carbamazepine on board, we don't know exactly by how much.

The most commonly used NOAC I'm seeing used in practice (with the exception of apixaban) is rivaroxaban. Unfortunately, this has the same interaction risk with carbamazepine as apixaban. This likely is not going to be a great option either.

CYP3A4 and P-glycoprotein Inhibitors

As discussed in the rivaroxaban section, inhibitors of CYP3A4 and P-glycoprotein can increase concentrations of apixaban and increase the risk of bleeding.

Over-The-Counter Medications and Supplements

I discussed St. John's Wort in the rivaroxaban section and it holds true that this should be avoided. This supplement is an inducer that can reduce the effectiveness of apixaban and increase the risk for a blood clot.

On the flip side, we do have numerous supplements and over-the-counter medications that can possibly increase the risk of bleeding. Ginger, garlic, and vitamin E supplements all have been associated with bleeding risk. I would say that these interactions are much less significant than a standard antiplatelet agent like aspirin or clopidogrel, but the evidence for any beneficial effects of these supplements isn't very solid. Turmeric is another supplement that I occasionally see utilized. In general, I encourage patients to avoid these supplements. If they are adamant about continuing to take these supplements, I definitely educate them about the potential cumulative risks.

Fish Oil is a supplement that has been controversial as far as antiplatelet and blood-thinning effects go. In general, I recommend avoiding the use of fish oil unless there is a good indication for the patient to be on it. In that situation, we can be a little extra careful and ensure that they are aware that there might be an exaggerated minor risk of bleed at the most.

When assessing supplements and their risks, it is also important to consider the dosing of the supplement. If patients are using standard over the counter dosing, the risks will likely tend to be lower. If you have patients that are inappropriately using high doses, they are really stepping in uncharted territory and it is hard to predict exactly what might happen and how significant a drug interaction or adverse effect might be because of an unusually high dose.

Assessment of pain is critical in patients taking anticoagulants. A good chunk of the population will begin taking over-the-counter medications prior to having their pain assessed by a medical provider. This means that many of them will be considering using NSAIDs like ibuprofen and naproxen. These meds should generally be avoided in patients on anticoagulation, but if they are used together it for sure should be done under medical supervision where we can help monitor and assess those risks with the patient.

Gemfibrozil

Statin Gemfibrozil Interaction

In most situations, gemfibrozil is not going to be the preferred agent in the management of hypertriglyceridemia. There appears to be a slightly lower risk of rhabdomyolysis with the use of fenofibrate. With that stated, you may run into patients who may be taking both gemfibrozil in combination with a statin. Let's lay out some strategies for dealing with this.

The first item to identify is if the patient is tolerating the combination. In most cases, if they are still on both agents, they are likely tolerating the combination. In this situation of good tolerability, there is a temptation to just leave the combination alone. That is not something I would generally prefer. Switching to fenofibrate would be a strong consideration and likely preferable in most situations.

Another item to consider is where are the triglyceride levels and do we actually need to treat them with gemfibrozil in addition to the statin. In many cases, it may be adequate to simply use a statin alone. Assessing for the risk of pancreatitis and how elevated the triglycerides are would be two important considerations.

Patient monitoring can be considered as well. Simply assessing the patient to identify if they are having signs and symptoms of myopathy is going to be important. If there is a question about tolerability and there is a strong desire to continue the combination, we can monitor CPK to ensure that we aren't running the risk of rhabdomyolysis.

Does an individual statin make a difference? US labeling of rosuvastatin may allow for concomitant use of gemfibrozil and rosuvastatin. However, it is recommended that the dose of rosuvastatin be limited to 10 mg/day. Depending upon what dose our patient is on and the cardiovascular risk, reducing the dose of rosuvastatin may not be appropriate which would lead us down the road of looking for an alternative to the gemfibrozil.

Gemfibrozil and Other Lipid Therapies

In addition to statins, there is a substantial risk of rhabdomyolysis with gemfibrozil in combination with other lipid-lowering therapies. Because of the similar classification and risk for overlapping adverse effects, gemfibrozil and fenofibrate would never be recommended to be used together. In addition, using ezetimibe in combination with gemfibrozil can increase the risk of rhabdomyolysis.

CYP2C8 Inhibition

Gemfibrozil has the potential to inhibit the enzyme CYP2C8. CYP2C8 is a major enzyme for drug metabolism, but there is one diabetes medication that can be impacted. By inhibiting CYP2C8, gemfibrozil can raise the concentrations of pioglitazone. Limiting the dose of pioglitazone to 15 mg would be an appropriate strategy. You'd also want to keep an eye out for pioglitazone adverse effects. The most common adverse effect to monitor for would be edema. Hypoglycemia would be concerning, particularly if a patient is receiving insulin or another oral agent that stimulates the release of insulin.

Montelukast is another agent that is occasionally used in the management of asthma and or allergies. Similar to pioglitazone, concentrations of montelukast can be significantly increased when used in combination with gemfibrozil.
In the setting of adverse effects from montelukast, it would be reasonable to reduce the dose or discontinue the gemfibrozil in an attempt to mitigate the risk of the interaction.

Hypoglycemia Risk

Gemfibrozil has the potential to interact with sulfonylureas and increase the risk of hypoglycemia. This potential interaction doesn't make the combination contraindicated, but it does make sense to be aware of the interaction and monitor the patient accordingly. Also, be aware of your patient's past medical history pertaining to hypoglycemia. If they have significant hypoglycemia episodes in the past or are at risk for serious negative outcomes from hypoglycemia events (i.e. elderly patients) it might be advisable to avoid sulfonylureas altogether in favor of an alternative diabetes medication.

In addition to the hypoglycemia risk with sulfonylureas, there is a contraindication to the use of gemfibrozil with repaglinide. Repaglinide can increase endogenous insulin production. Gemfibrozil can substantially raise the concentrations of repaglinide. Significant increases in repaglinide concentrations can be a major cause for concern when considering hypoglycemia. In clinical practice, repaglinide is virtually never utilized, but there is an odd chance you may see it.

Ezetimibe

Ezetimibe is generally not considered near as effective at lowering cholesterol compared to statin therapy. However, it is generally considered a little more tolerable and may have less frequent and significant drug interactions compared to statins.

Fibrate Risk

As discussed in the gemfibrozil section, using ezetimibe in combination with gemfibrozil is not recommended due to the risk of rhabdomyolysis. To a lesser extent, there may be a small, increased risk of myopathy and rhabdomyolysis when fenofibrate derivatives are used in combination with ezetimibe.

Binding Interaction – Bile Acid Sequestrants

Bile acid sequestrants aren't commonly used for hyperlipidemia, but occasionally you may seem them used for unexplained diarrhea management. The potential of bile acid sequestrants like cholestyramine to bind up drugs is real and concerning. With ezetimibe, there is a risk of reduced absorption and clinical activity when cholestyramine is used near the administration time of ezetimibe.

Digoxin

P-glycoprotein Inhibition

Digoxin concentration is significantly impacted by P-glycoprotein activity. Inhibitors of P-glycoprotein will likely cause digoxin concentrations to rise while any drug that may induce P-glycoprotein may cause concentrations to fall. There are a significant number of drugs that can affect P-glycoprotein. Some examples of medications that may inhibit P-glycoprotein include some of the azole antifungals, mirabegron, colchicine, and amiodarone. Below is a case scenario with the use of amiodarone, canagliflozin, and digoxin.

Amiodarone Digoxin

A 67 year old male has a past medical history of hypertension, atrial fibrillation, CHF, and osteoarthritis. He has had numerous issues with his cardiac status and it has led him to frequent physician visits, including the involvement of a cardiologist.

This gentleman has been on digoxin 250 mcg daily with digoxin levels around the 0.8 mark. He has had no symptoms of toxicity. Due to the cardiologist's findings, he feels it is appropriate to add amiodarone to this patient's regimen.

Of course, the amiodarone digoxin interaction is one you need to be aware of. Amiodarone can significantly raise the concentration of digoxin in the body potentially leading to digoxin toxicity. The proposed mechanism of this interaction involves amiodarone's potential to inhibit the action of P-glycoprotein. By inhibiting P-glycoprotein in the GI tract, this prevents the body from pumping digoxin back into the gut for elimination. Ultimately this is going to lead to an elevation in the concentrations of digoxin.

A reduction in the dose of digoxin will likely be required in this situation with a new start of amiodarone. The cardiologist would hopefully be all over this drug interaction, but you should be aware of it as well. In the event a dose reduction is not made, you must monitor this patient very carefully. Monitoring for signs of digoxin toxicity like nausea, vomiting, weight loss, alterations in heart rate, CNS changes, and visual changes is critical to ensure patient safety from the risk of this interaction.

Digoxin Potassium Relationship

Individuals with low potassium may be more susceptible to possible digoxin toxicity. Why is that? Potassium and digoxin bind to the same location on the ATPase pump. If there is less potassium to compete for this binding site, there is the potential for more digoxin to be able to bind in that location. It is very important to recognize this risk as well as medications that may affect potassium levels.

What drugs can affect potassium levels? In many cases, digoxin is used in the management of congestive heart failure. In congestive heart failure, there is a high utilization of diuretics (especially loop diuretics) which can significantly reduce potassium levels and potentially increase the risk of digoxin toxicity as described above. Close monitoring of renal function and potassium levels are very important when appropriately using digoxin. In addition to loop diuretics, thiazide diuretics can also lower potassium levels and would increase the risk of digoxin toxicity.

Cardiac Activity

Digoxin is well known to slow down the heart rate and contribute to bradycardia. We need to be careful with the use of agents that can have additive effects. Drugs like beta-blockers and non-dihydropyridine calcium channel blockers can increase the risk of bradycardia. When avoidance of this combination is not possible, we need to ensure these patients are closely monitored and that dose adjustments are made if the heart rate is dropping too significantly.

Renal Function

It is critical to remember that worsening renal function can lead to rising concentrations of digoxin. Be sure to recognize medications that may increase the risk of renal impairment. If reductions in kidney function go on for any significant amount of time, it can lead to an accumulation of digoxin for any patient on this medication.

Propylene Glycol Risks – Metronidazole

There are numerous IV medications that contain propylene glycol. It is critical to recognize that there is a risk with these medications as metronidazole can cause a disulfiram reaction with any product that contains this component. Digoxin is one of the medications that can contain this component. Other medications that can potentially contain propylene glycol include diazepam, phenytoin, and lorazepam. Common symptoms of the disulfiram drug reaction include headache, flushing, nausea, and vomiting.

Nitroglycerin and Isosorbide Mononitrate

Nitroglycerin and PDE5 Inhibitors

Every now and again, I will run into patients with both angina as well as erectile dysfunction. The nitroglycerin sildenafil drug interaction is one that should be taken seriously. Coadministration of these medications should be avoided. Mechanistically, vasodilation is much more likely to occur due to this interaction. Vasodilation happens because there is an increase in cyclic GMP (cGMP). Nitroglycerin works on the front end by creating and facilitating the release of more cGMP. Phosphodiesterase-5 inhibitors work on the backend by preventing the breakdown of cGMP. The possible end result of taking these together is very significant hypotension.

Using sildenafil as our example, here are a few considerations I think of when trying to figure out how to manage this drug interaction.

Is the sildenafil really necessary? Many patients may be on drugs that contribute to erectile dysfunction and those should be assessed/reassessed. Certain antidepressants and antihypertensives are a couple of classic examples of medications that could contribute to erectile dysfunction. Make sure the patients' other medications aren't causing the problem. With antidepressants and antihypertensives, it isn't always easy to transition these to another agent, but it is worthwhile to ask the patient about this if other options haven't been explored.

How often is the patient needing nitroglycerin? If the patient was prescribed nitroglycerin 10 years ago and has never used it, the likelihood of coadministration is very low. As long as the patient understands the interaction and is comfortable with the situation, it is likely ok.

How often is the sildenafil being used? I've met with numerous patients that have sildenafil (or other PDE-5) on their medication list, but they haven't used the medication in years. In that situation, stopping the sildenafil may be a possibility.

If a patient believes that they can manage both, obviously we have to do our best job of educating the patient that coadministration should be avoided. It is important to note that there should be a longer separation period than 24 hours for a PDE-5 inhibitor that has a longer half-life. It is recommended to avoid coadministration of tadalafil and nitrates within 48 hours of one another.

Additive Effects

Because of the potential and likely the goal of using nitrates for their antianginal and blood pressure-lowering effect, this can be both beneficial and detrimental. If blood pressure drops too low, our patient may be at risk for falls and dizziness. Be aware of other blood pressure-lowering medications and use nitrates cautiously when starting the medication to ensure it is well tolerated. In the setting of chest pain or ACS, we may have to use PRN nitroglycerin and monitor the blood pressure closely. Educating the patient to be aware of the possibility of low blood pressure is very important as well. When a nitrate has been started or increased, have the patient be really careful with position changes (i.e. sitting to standing) to allow the body to adapt and get adequate perfusion to the brain.

It is also important to note the difference in pharmacokinetics for nitroglycerin sublingual compared to isosorbide mononitrate. The sublingual nitroglycerin has a very quick onset and also a very short half-life. The likelihood of the blood pressure-lowering effects occurring hours after administration of nitroglycerin SL is low. The most likely timeframe for dizziness and low blood pressure would be within the first 20-30 minutes of administration. Isosorbide mononitrate has a half-life of several hours. The potential for hypotension could linger most of the day following a dose of isosorbide mononitrate.

There are countless drugs that can lower blood pressure. ACE inhibitors, ARBs, alpha-blockers, calcium channel blockers, diuretics, beta-blockers, antipsychotics, clonidine, levodopa, and dopamine agonists are a few examples.

CYP3A4 Inhibition

Nitroglycerin sublingual is not likely to be impacted by CYP3A4 enzyme alterations. However, isosorbide mononitrate and isosorbide dinitrate concentrations may be increased by CYP3A4 inhibitors. Keep an eye out for drugs like fluconazole, erythromycin, verapamil, diltiazem, and the supplement grapefruit juice. Hypotension would be more likely if these drugs are used in combination. This may be especially true with verapamil and diltiazem as they can lower blood pressure themselves in addition to the potential to raise the concentration of the nitrate.

Alcohol and Nitrates

It is best to avoid alcohol. Alcohol can have vasodilation type effects and increase the likelihood of flushing. When used in combination with nitrates, alcohol could have added vasodilatory effects leading to a lower blood pressure.

Amiodarone

QTC Prolongation and Amiodarone

When you think of amiodarone, we have to think about QTc prolongation. Addressing QTc prolongation drug interactions has always been a challenging topic for me. These drug interactions are really hard to know what to do with. Problems arising from these interactions rarely happen, but obviously QTc prolongation can increase the risk of incredibly serious events like Torsades de points. Here are a few thoughts on this topic:

Assess the risk of the medication being added, started, or changed. Amiodarone interactions are very notable. When adding other medications to amiodarone that also prolong the QT interval, proceed in a cautious manner.

In patients at risk of QTc prolongation, are other agents acceptable? Example: In the situation where we are treating an infection with antibiotic therapy, can we avoid quinolones or macrolides? Both classes of medications can prolong the QT interval, but we may have many appropriate alternatives depending upon the infection we are trying to treat.

Minimize dose and/or duration where possible. As far as minimizing dose, citalopram is the classic example that has numerous QTc prolongation drug interactions, amiodarone included. If we can taper down and ensure that the patient is at the lowest dose possible, this is closest to the ideal scenario of not using a QTc prolonging drug altogether. Looking at minimizing the duration of therapy for antibiotics or ondansetron are two good examples where maybe we can get away with shorter treatment durations.

EKG monitoring. In patients who have known risk factors and must be on medications that can prolong the QT interval, EKG monitoring is an important tool to assess and minimize the risk of potentially dangerous consequences.

Keep an eye out for electrolyte imbalances. Magnesium and potassium are two big ones that come to mind when we talk about potential cardiac problems.

Assessing that these levels are within the normal range can be an important factor to reduce the risk of potential cardiac problems from QTc prolongation and drug interactions.

Here's a list (not all-inclusive) of some common medications that will come up as potential drug interactions with amiodarone for QTc prolongation risk:
- Antiarrhythmics
- Sotalol, quinidine, procainamide, dofetilide
- TCAs
- Amitriptyline, nortriptyline, doxepin, imipramine
- SSRIs (particularly citalopram)
- Antibiotics
- Quinolones (levofloxacin)
- Macrolides (erythromycin, clarithromycin)

CYP3A4 Effects

Amiodarone is metabolized by CYP3A4. This means that any drug that inhibits or induces CYP3A4 will potentially alter the concentrations of amiodarone. This could lead to alterations in cardiac contractility and lead to the risk of worsening arrhythmia. In addition, toxicity may be more likely in those patients who are taking a CYP3A4 inhibitor. Examples of CYP3A4 inhibitors that would increase concentrations of amiodarone include HIV drugs like ritonavir and cobicistat, many of the systemic azole antifungals, and macrolides like clarithromycin. If amiodarone is necessary as it will likely be, finding alternatives to these agents would be important. It is also critical to educate and assess patients about the risks of grapefruit juice and its potential to raise amiodarone concentrations.

Inducers of CYP3A4 would lower concentrations of amiodarone. Carbamazepine, phenytoin, and rifampin are three common examples of medications that would lower amiodarone concentrations.

Amiodarone also can inhibit CYP3A4. This means that many drugs that are broken down by this enzyme can have increased concentrations. When cyclosporine is used in the setting of immunosuppression for a transplant patient, maintaining therapeutic levels and avoid toxicity is critical. By inhibiting CYP3A4, amiodarone can upset a previously stable level and increase the risk of toxicity. Also, consider that many commonly used statins may be broken down by CYP3A4. Simvastatin, lovastatin, and atorvastatin concentrations may be increased when amiodarone is initiated or increased.

Bradycardia

Amiodarone is an antiarrhythmic medication and it can increase the likelihood of bradycardia. This is especially true when used in combination with other medications that can cause bradycardia. The use of beta-blockers and/or non-dihydropyridine calcium channel blockers in combination with amiodarone can significantly increase the risk for bradycardia. Close monitoring of pulse while making changes in these medications would be important to assess.

Amiodarone and Thyroid Function

Patients who take thyroid replacement should be aware of amiodarone and the potential it has to alter thyroid function. While hyperthyroidism is reported in the literature, it is much more common for amiodarone to oppose the effects of thyroid supplementation. It can do this in the presence of thyroid supplementation or in patients who are not currently taking thyroid supplementation. Be aware of this potential drug interaction in those who are taking amiodarone and levothyroxine as well as those patients who are not on levothyroxine or another form of thyroid replacement. Here's a case example of a patient where amiodarone caused hypothyroidism.

An 88 y/o with a history of depressive type symptoms was placed on an antidepressant to manage symptoms shortly after admission to a long term care facility.

This particular patient was trialed on Zoloft (sertraline) and then transitioned to Cymbalta (duloxetine), neither of which made a significant difference in symptoms. This patient continued to have ongoing symptoms of depression despite antidepressant therapy.

Hypothyroid symptoms can often overlap/mimic signs of depression and this is a scenario I've seen play out several times. What was of note, was that the patient was on chronic amiodarone for an arrhythmia. Amiodarone has many unique side effects one of which is it can affect thyroid function. It was requested that a TSH be checked to monitor for this unique side effect of amiodarone. TSH lab work was done and elevated at about 30 indicating hypothyroidism – normal range is approximately 0.5-6 depending upon the lab. Synthroid was initiated and the symptoms of "depression" started to improve allowing for discontinuation of the Cymbalta (duloxetine).

QTC Prolongation Case Example

Here's a case scenario of possible medication-induced QTc prolongation and some thoughts as to what I might do about it. The medication list includes:

- Amitriptyline 150 mg once daily
- Geodon 80 mg BID
- Metformin 500 mg BID
- Ondansetron 8 mg TID PRN
- Gabapentin 300 mg TID
- Ativan 1 mg daily
- Glipizide 5 mg daily
- Losartan 100 mg daily
- Aspirin 81 mg daily
- Atorvastatin 10 mg daily
- Aripiprazole 10 mg daily

An EKG was performed and the QTc, when checked, was 523. The patient has not had cardiac concerns in the past. When assessing possible medication-induced QTc prolongation, I would want to know if an EKG was checked in the past and if so, how much has it changed/increased since the last time it was checked. With this high of a result, reducing some medications would be likely appropriate. If there has been a change in QTc, it would also be nice to know the timing of that change and if it correlates with the addition of any medications.

The first thing I would look at is the ondansetron and if that is being used. It is known to contribute to QTc prolongation.

Antipsychotics are another medication class that should be looked at. Finding a way to avoid using two antipsychotics would be a good idea. This is likely a patient that has a very substantial mental health history and that needs to be reviewed. Ziprasidone (Geodon) is likely a little higher risk than the aripiprazole as far as QTc prolongation goes.

Amitriptyline should also be looked at as far as potential for QTc prolongation. In a scenario like this, some tough decisions will likely have to be made by the team in relation to the psych medications.

Anticholinergics – GI Ulceration

One of the important adverse effects to recognize from anticholinergic medications is that they slow down the GI tract. This can impact the transition of medications through the gut. There have been instances of the gut slowing down so much that slow-release potassium tablets can stick to the intestinal wall. If this occurs, it can cause significant damage to the mucosal layer of the gut and lead to gastrointestinal ulceration.

The major question you should consider is how "anticholinergic" is a medication. This will help allow you to assess the clinical significance and how much concern you should have for this drug interaction. If you have a patient on high dose diphenhydramine for itching, a TCA like amitriptyline for depression, and oxybutynin for urinary incontinence, your patient will be at much greater risk for this to occur. If your patient is on an inhaled anticholinergic that will have minimal absorption and systemic impact, GI ulceration is much less likely to happen. I discuss ipratropium's risk as well as challenges in utilizing drug interaction screening programs below.

Avoiding and reducing the anticholinergic burden is one way to avoid or minimize the risk of this interaction. Another way to reduce the risk of this from happening is to change the patient to a dosage formulation that is liquid. The risk is really from the tablet or capsule sticking to the lining of the GI tract. If we use liquid potassium, we can avoid this risk altogether. Unfortunately, liquid potassium may not taste very good to many patients. Some of the tablets may be able to be dissolved into water. Klor-Con M tab may be dissolved in 4 ounces of water. This takes a couple of minutes to accomplish but may mitigate the GI ulceration risk.

Patient education will also be a factor in trying to reduce the potential for this effect. Encouraging the patient to take potassium with a significant amount of water may also help aid in allowing adequate flow through the esophagus. This can also aid in the dissolution process. You may need to be careful in patients who have fluid restrictions, but otherwise, most patients should not have an issue with this and is something they can easily do to help reduce the risk of this complication.

I do want to emphasize that I have encountered many situations where potassium supplements are no longer necessary. In some situations (i.e. when a diuretic has been discontinued), it is possible that we could discontinue the potassium supplement and avoid the possibility of this interaction altogether.

Ipratropium and Potassium Supplements

Is there really a standard way to deal with drug interactions? My answer, you cannot treat them all the same. I see all sorts of different faxes from different pharmacies as well as notifications from electronic health software in nursing homes, home cares, or assisted livings warning of drug interactions. It's really just weird and a waste of time in many cases. I cannot recall one fax from a pharmacy or other institution about a patient taking an NSAID with warfarin. Not one, and trust me, I've seen these drugs used together numerous times. Maybe the individual looking at this assumes the prescriber is aware of this? This is one of the hallmark drug interactions and is on many top ten lists for most concerning interaction and I can't recall ever seeing a single fax?

I once saw a drug interaction alert faxed to a physician. It was regarding the inhaled anticholinergic (ipratropium) with solid oral dosage forms of potassium. It was of the highest severity. The thought is that the anticholinergic effects slow GI motility and the potassium can cause an ulcer or damage the GI tract. Really??? I went to look up this interaction and Lexi-comp lists it as an "X" – the highest severity. Next, I looked up the amount absorbed into the body from inhaled ipratropium. Systemic absorption of ipratropium is considered "negligible". If it's negligible, how is this an interaction, much less an interaction of highest severity? A computer program cannot provide common sense. These programs are a tool, not a brain, and I do have a concern that some healthcare professionals may expect their program to save them. We can all miss important interactions, and computer programs can help us flag interactions, but we need to give a thoughtful clinical review of an interaction before dispensing, prescribing, or administering a medication.

Hyperkalemia Risk

One of the dangers of polypharmacy is the potential for drug interactions. While it may seem obvious to most reading this book that potassium supplements can increase the risk for hyperkalemia, I have seen it missed. When I have seen this overlooked, in the majority of cases, it has been because the patient is taking other medications that increase the risk of hyperkalemia and they have a medication list that is generally multiple pages.

Be aware of potassium levels when altering doses of other drugs that can impact potassium levels. ACE inhibitors, ARBs, and spironolactone are the most commonly used agents that can raise potassium levels.

Vitamin D

Hypercalcemia Risk

From a mechanism of action standpoint, recall that vitamin D increases calcium primarily by increasing GI absorption of calcium. While hypercalcemia is not a common occurrence under normal over-the-counter supplemental doses of vitamin D, it should be considered in patients who may have a chronic issue with hypercalcemia, or in those who may be at higher risk for hypercalcemia. Those who may be at higher risk for hypercalcemia include those who may have cumulative drug interactions that raise calcium levels. Vitamin D in combination with patients who are taking lots of calcium carbonate for heartburn may carry an added risk for hypercalcemia. Also, recall that thiazide diuretics can raise calcium levels as well. Be aware of these combinations and monitor calcium levels to ensure that we are not putting our patients at risk for hypercalcemia. I generally look at this risk a little more closely if I have patients who are on unusually high doses of agents that can cause hypercalcemia, have an elevated level or have a history of hypercalcemia.

Duplicate Therapy

Patients are often unaware of what their supplements actually contain. There is a relatively low risk for vitamin D toxicity in most patients, but in those who may inadvertently take numerous supplements with vitamin D as a component, this can have a cumulative effect. Recall that vitamin D is a fat-soluble vitamin that can accumulate in the body.

Aluminum Interaction

Much like vitamin D can increase the absorption of calcium, it can also increase the risk of aluminum toxicity. I have not found that many patients use aluminum hydroxide as an antacid type agent, but be aware that patients who take vitamin D may aid in the systemic

84

absorption of aluminum. In addition, sucralfate, a prescription GI medication used for heartburn type symptoms also contains aluminum. Vitamin D can raise the systemic absorption of aluminum in this product as well. In the odd chance that a patient is taking this combination, it would be easiest to select another GI medication. Patients who may be at higher risk of aluminum accumulation include patients who have renal dysfunction.

Reduced Absorption of Vitamin D

As I mentioned earlier, vitamin D is a fat-soluble vitamin. There are medications that can reduce or prevent the absorption of fat-soluble vitamins. Mineral oil is an over the counter agent that when taken orally can help manage constipation. I would strongly discourage its use, especially in the elderly, for this purpose as it can cause significant complications if aspirated. However, if patients are taking it over-the-counter chronically, there is potential for deficiency of fat-soluble vitamins like vitamin D. Orlistat is another medication that can impair its absorption. Orlistat is a medication that can be used for weight loss. It essentially blocks the absorption of fat in the gut so it is removed from the body in the stool. With that removal of fat, fat-soluble vitamins can be contained within and absorption impaired.

Vitamin D Deficiency

Dilantin (phenytoin) is probably one of the dirtiest drugs but may be necessary as it treats an obviously serious condition (seizures). It has many clinical quirks that you need to be aware of. A 72 year old female with a long history of seizures was on a maintenance dose of 200 mg twice daily. Seizures were well managed and patient displayed no symptoms of phenytoin toxicity with a total phenytoin level of 12. (Remember the clinical quirks about phenytoin levels especially if your patient is displaying symptoms of toxicity!) This particular patient was just recently admitted to the hospital for a wrist fracture, and it was discovered that she had osteoporosis. Upon this discovery, the provider ordered a vitamin D level to assess if and how much supplementation they felt was necessary. The level came back at 6. (normal is 30-100 in most labs) Why was this level so low? – Long term phenytoin can cause/worsen vitamin D deficiency. The patient was started on a Vitamin D supplement.

Binding Interactions

With the use of iron supplementation, the major drug interactions you need to be aware of are binding interactions. There are numerous cases where iron can bind a drug in the GI tract and reduce the absorption of that medication. Keep in mind that this is only for iron preparations that are absorbed through the GI tract. This does not include IV iron. Levodopa, levothyroxine, and bisphosphonates are three medications whose absorption can be reduced on account of oral iron preparations in the gut.

There is a relatively new medication that can be used for the treatment of influenza. Baloxavir can help relieve symptoms and reduce the length of time it takes to recover from influenza. This drug is contraindicated with iron as iron can reduce concentrations by binding up the drug and reduce the overall efficacy.

Antibiotics like quinolones and tetracycline derivates can be fairly tightly bound to iron and substantial reductions in blood concentrations can result. When we are treating infections, we run the risk of treatment failure. Here's a case scenario where this interaction occurred:

A 44 year old male has a history of respiratory issues. He is diagnosed at the clinic with pneumonia. Levaquin (oral) was initiated for a 10 day period.

Current medication list includes:
- Advair 250/50 twice daily
- Albuterol as needed
- Hydrochlorothiazide 25 mg daily
- Ferrous Sulfate 325 mg twice daily
- Prilosec 20 mg daily

Day 7 of 10 for the Levaquin course and the patient is not improving. He presents to the clinic for a reassessment of pneumonia and requests a different medication. A Z-pak (azithromycin for 5 days) is prescribed and within 3-5 days the patient begins feeling much better with a full resolution of pneumonia following treatment with azithromycin.

So, what happened? We can only speculate, but I've got three major points that I think could've been the problem.

- Assessment of adherence is critical with antibiotics and any medication for that matter – that is where I would start.
- Resistance to antibiotics is a significant problem and could be at play here.
- I've seen this happen several times, and I think it might lead to failure more often then we realize, especially with quinolone antibiotics. The iron and Levaquin drug interaction is well-known, but does slip through the cracks, especially with polypharmacy complicating things. Iron can significantly block the absorption of Levaquin leading to low concentrations in the blood and potentially low enough to cause the failure of treatment. Again, we can only speculate in this case scenario, but this is an interaction you should be aware of and frequently assess for use of products with iron, calcium, and magnesium which can all bind up quinolone antibiotics.

Acid Suppressing Drugs

One unique pearl about oral iron absorption is that absorption increases as the pH of the stomach decreases. It is important to be aware of drugs that can raise the pH as any patient who is taking antacid medications could have impaired iron absorption. Classic examples of medications that reduce stomach acid include PPIs, H2 blockers, and over the counter antacids. We can monitor iron levels to help assess if iron absorption is adequate. If we are utilizing iron supplements for anemia, we will also likely see a response in the hemoglobin. Avoiding coadministration with antacids can potentially help, but H2 blockers and PPIs tend to have a longer duration of action. Ensuring that we are using the minimum effective dose or possibly discontinuing (where appropriate) these medications for those patients who need iron replacement are two potential considerations. IV iron does have some risks and is expensive, but for someone who is not absorbing an adequate amount of iron through the gut, this is a consideration.

Folic Acid

Sulfasalazine

Sulfasalazine has the potential to reduce folic acid absorption and increase the risk of deficiency. Important monitoring parameters include assessing for folic acid deficiency. Folic acid is an important

87

component of red blood cell production. Checking a CBC and watching for signs and symptoms of anemia can help manage this potential risk with sulfasalazine.

Phenytoin

Folic acid uniquely has the potential to affect the concentrations of phenytoin. As you can imagine, a lowering of phenytoin concentrations can increase the risk of our patient having a seizure. It isn't clear how exactly this drug interaction happens, but it may be due to folic acid being a necessary component in the enzymatic process of breaking down phenytoin. Closely monitor patients who have started taking folic acid and who are on phenytoin for the risk of seizures or lower concentrations.

Taking Advantage of a Drug Interaction - Methotrexate

Methotrexate is a medication used in oncology (as well as rheumatologic disorders). In oncology, it ultimately inhibits DNA synthesis by preventing dihydrofolate reductase action which can cause death in cancer (as well as normal) cells. Leucovorin is a form of folic acid. Leucovorin is used in oncology to help replace folate stores and ultimately will reduce the effectiveness of methotrexate. This is strategically done to try to prevent methotrexate toxicity.

Taking Advantage of a Drug Interaction – Fluorouracil

With the use of fluorouracil, leucovorin does the opposite of what it does compared with methotrexate. Leucovorin will help stabilize thymidylate synthase and facilitate binding with fluorouracil. This aid in binding fluorouracil will lead to an increase in the effectiveness of the oncology agent.

Vitamin B12 (oral)

Metformin

Vitamin B12 supplements are used by many patients. Some patients will take them on their own without any evidence of deficiency and some patients can have symptoms of B12 deficiency. There are possible serious complications from substantial B12 deficiency. Metformin can cause reduced absorption from the GI tract. We should be aware of this potential reduction and the fact that metformin can oppose the supplementation that we are trying to help their deficiency with. With enough supplementation, we can usually overcome this effect. To keep tabs on this interaction, we can continue to assess the risk for anemia by monitoring hemoglobin.

It is also important to note that there are special populations where this interaction may be exacerbated. In patients who've had gastric bypass or other GI surgeries that may reduce the absorption of B12, we need to be especially aware of the risk for deficiency. In addition to patients with an altered GI tract, elderly patients can be deficient in intrinsic factor which is a necessary component for proper gut absorption of B12. Be aware that these patients may be extra sensitive to drugs that may impair oral absorption of B12.

PPIs

PPIs are widely used in clinical practice and there is potential for these drugs to impair the absorption of B12. By blocking gastric acid production, this can reduce the production of pepsin. Pepsin is very important in the breakdown of protein and ultimately the release of vitamin B12 from that protein. Be aware that PPIs can increase the risk of B12 deficiency. Monitoring levels and assessing patients for signs and symptoms of B12 deficiency is critical in patients taking drugs that can impair or inhibit B12 absorption.

Colchicine

Colchicine is a medication that can be used in the management of gout. Much like PPIs and metformin, it can alter the absorption of B12 and make deficiency more likely. Appropriate monitoring and assessment for B12 deficiency signs and symptoms are critical.

Omega-3 Fatty Acids (Fish Oil)

Bleeding Risk

Many patients take over the counter fish oil. Fish oil has been associated with having antiplatelet activity, but the clinical significance of the severity of this effect is still debated. When we have clinical questions where we don't know what study to believe, I recommend proceeding with caution. The theoretical risk with the use of fish oil would be an increase in bleeding. As far as drug interactions are concerned, we need to be aware of patients who may be already taking medications that increase this risk. Pay close attention to those receiving anticoagulation, NSAIDs, and antiplatelet medication. If there are concerns with blood loss, excessive bruising or other signs that may indicate thinning of the blood, avoiding fish oil would be my recommendation.

In addition to monitoring for bleed risk, I would ensure that we have good evidence as to why we are using the fish oil. In the management of cholesterol, management with over-the-counter dosing fish oil is likely not enough to be an effective way to help our patients. Most patients I have worked with have said that they started taking it because they heard that it is good for their heart health or health in general. In patients who have bleeding risks and no indication to take the fish oil, I would generally recommend discontinuing the fish oil.

Calcium

Binding Interactions

Calcium is well known to bind up many medications and risk the effects of low drug concentrations. This can lead to treatment failure. Quinolones, tetracycline antibiotics, baloxavir, mycophenolate, sotalol, and levothyroxine are all drugs that can be substantially impacted by coadministration with calcium. It is going to be rare that patients are using calcium for anything other than bone health. In patients who are needing a short term medication that is bound by calcium, it may be easiest to hold the calcium dose for a period of time. On occasion, the drugs that interact with calcium may be dosed a couple of times per day and calcium itself may be dosed twice per day. In this situation, it is difficult to get the timing of all these doses correctly which makes simply holding the medication desirable.

In the setting of chronic medication, we need to assess how the patient is taking the medications and what the timing of each one is. We also need to consider if the patient has been taking their medications in a consistent manner for a long time. If they have been taking their levothyroxine close to the same time as their calcium but their thyroid levels are within the normal range, we are likely going to recommend that they remain consistent with the timing of administration. We would also recommend that they keep getting their routine TSH done to ensure that everything remains stable.

Allopurinol is another medication that can potentially have concentrations reduced by calcium supplementation. If the patient is having gout flares or needing escalating doses of allopurinol to keep uric acid low, taking calcium with allopurinol may compound this concern. While we don't typically check an allopurinol level, we can certainly recognize this interaction and review the timing of administration in patients who are struggling to get their uric acid and gout symptoms under control.

Reduced Absorption

Iron requires an acidic environment to be effectively absorbed. This may not happen if a patient is taking calcium carbonate on a routine basis or close to the same time as their iron. Be sure to assess the use of "Tums" or other heartburn relieving medications. This also stresses the importance of asking about over-the-counter medications and supplements that the patient may be taking on their own. In addition, we can recognize patients who are not responding to iron therapy by assessing their iron stores (i.e. ferritin).

Calcium Overload

Rarely I have seen situations where patients are taking too much calcium with other agents that can elevate calcium levels. Vitamin D and thiazide diuretics can cause hypercalcemia and this in combination with frequent use of calcium supplements can put a patient at a very high risk for hypercalcemia. The situation where this is most common is in a patient who is "popping" calcium carbonate like candy for management of heartburn and GI upset. Keep an eye out for this if your patient's calcium level is abnormally high. Calcium levels are easily assessed by checking lab work.

Additive Effects

Constipation is a well-known concern with the use of calcium. Elderly patients can be especially at risk for constipation due to polypharmacy. Recognize other medications that may have a cumulative effect on this symptom. Opioids, anticholinergic medications, and calcium channel blockers are common examples of medications that could exacerbate constipation. When we combine multiple medications that can cause this adverse effect, we run an increased risk of creating problems.

Magnesium

Binding Interactions

Much like calcium and iron supplements, oral magnesium can be the cause of numerous binding interactions. Tetracycline antibiotics like doxycycline and minocycline can be bound by magnesium and their concentrations reduced. Other medications include quinolones, levothyroxine, mycophenolate, and gabapentin. With quinolones and the tetracyclines, we certainly need to worry about treatment failure. When looking at the levothyroxine interaction, we can monitor TSH to ensure that the levothyroxine dose is still adequate and being absorbed. Consistency and having euthyroid lab work is the primary objective with levothyroxine. With the use of mycophenolate, the indication can make a significant difference in how concerned we are about the interaction. If mycophenolate is being used in the setting of transplantation, it is essential to recognize that this drug interaction could lead to devastating consequences in the form of low concentrations and possible organ rejection. The gabapentin magnesium interaction is probably less concerning than mycophenolate in the setting of neuropathy treatment. The risk is an increase in pain. While this isn't desirable, it is likely not going to be as concerning as a possible organ rejection.

With all of these interactions, I'd assess if the magnesium is necessary. Many patients will take this supplement on their own to manage leg cramps and other ailments. If the patient wants to continue to take the magnesium or if it is deemed necessary to maintain levels, then you must look at the timing of administration and attempt to give the magnesium a couple of hours after the interacting medication.

Alcohol

Clinical Considerations

Throughout the book, I have discussed numerous drug interactions relating to the use of alcohol by patients. One of the most challenging questions I get asked by patients is "Can I use alcohol with my medications?" It is such a loaded question. Here are a few of my thoughts when patients ask me this.

How much are we talking about? It is near impossible to tell how much alcohol the patient is talking about when they ask this question. Then, do we believe what they are saying, or are they being conservative in their assessment of how much they will drink? The patient likely doesn't know this answer for sure. This is the million-dollar question that is really hard to pin down.

Are they an elderly patient and at risk for falls? Alcohol can be a substantial contributing factor to falls, disinhibition, confusion, and poor judgment. Drug combinations, pharmacokinetics, and pharmacodynamics can certainly change in the elderly and may place this patient population at a higher risk of problems. Not to mention that typically the elderly are on more medications with more chronic health conditions.

Which medications are they taking? Some medications are definitely worse than others as far as potential interactions with alcohol. A few common examples of meds that may be more concerning (this is definitely not an all-inclusive list!)
1. Metronidazole
2. Benzodiazepines
3. Psychotropic medications
4. Opioids
5. Other sedatives/hypnotics

What conditions do they have? Having kidney disease and problems with dehydration may complicate this. Factor in the potential for using diuretics, NSAIDs, and/or ACE Inhibitors and the alcohol may exacerbate a potential dehydration scenario. Do they have liver impairment? If so, what drugs are they taking combined with alcohol that may enhance the risk for hepatotoxicity?

Do you think the patient might have an underlying problem with substance abuse? Chronic alcohol use can lead to a substantial amount of medical problems.

Identifying patients at risk for alcohol abuse for further assessment and getting them any help they might need is an important part of our job as healthcare professionals.

Once I've looked up any potential interactions with alcohol, these are some of the clinical questions I assess when a patient asks me if it is ok to use alcohol with their medication.

St. John's Wort

CYP3A4 Inducer

St. John's Wort is a notorious supplement in the healthcare community. One of the reasons it is so problematic is that it can induce the action of CYP3A4. CYP3A4 is responsible for the breakdown of hundreds of drugs. When St. John's Wort is added to a patient's medication regimen, you can likely bet that it will lower the concentration and clinical effects of at least some of the medications that the patient is taking. Anticoagulants, antiarrhythmics, certain statins, antifungal agents, HIV medications, and some antibiotics are a few of the major drug interactions that you need to be aware of when using this medication.

So, what would you say if a patient asked you, "Should I take St. John's Wort?" My gut screams no! However, we need to take everything into account before blindly saying no. Here are a few things I would consider before deciding on whether or not I would be ok with a patient taking this supplement.

- What do they want to take it for? Figuring out what the indication is would be step one. I would initially suspect they would want it for depression, but you don't know unless you ask.
- What's been tried? I'm going to assume most patients would ask about it for depression. Looking back at past medical history and figuring out what medications have been tried may provide you some insight as to why they want to use an herbal supplement with tons of medication interactions. If they have failed numerous other traditional prescription therapy medications, you could understand that they may be disheartened.
- What other drugs are they on? If this is a patient on 10+ medications or more, you're asking for more trouble than it is likely worth.
- How strongly does the patient feel about it? If it was merely an idea from a friend or relative, you can likely explain some of the risks associated with St. John's Wort and why you think an alternative is more appropriate.
- Is the patient willing/capable of being their own advocate and telling every healthcare professional they encounter that they are on St. John's Wort? This will be incredibly important whenever they are prescribed new medications because herbal supplements are often overlooked or not asked about.

Again, even if I liked all the responses from these questions, I would still be very apprehensive about a patient using this supplement.

P-glycoprotein Inducer

In addition to the action on CYP3A4, St. John's Wort can also induce P-glycoprotein. We discussed the implications of altering the function of P-glycoprotein in the Non-dihydropyridine calcium channel blocker section. In the majority of situations, a P-glycoprotein inducer like St. John's Wort will negatively impact serum concentrations of drugs.

Serotonergic Effects

If you can recall that patients are likely going to take St. John's Wort for the indication of depression, this should also jog your memory that it can impact serotonin. By impacting the activity of serotonin, patients may be at risk for serotonin syndrome if they are taking other agents that have serotonergic activity.

Blood Pressure Lowering Effect

Alpha-blockers are well known for their activity in managing BPH symptoms. They are also well known for helping to manage low blood pressure. Alpha-blockers are virtually never a first-line blood pressure medication when being strictly used for that purpose. The most common situation where non-selective alpha-blockers are used is in a patient who has a duplicate indication for them. One of the major reasons that they are not used first-line in hypertension is because they can cause significant drops in blood pressure. This is especially true when a patient first starts taking an alpha-blocker.

Be aware of patients who are taking other medications that can cause blood pressure lowering effects. I think we have outlined this pretty well in the hypertension section. Patient awareness and education are critical with this class of medication. Most of the time we will recommend that these medications be taken at night right before sleep so if there is that risk of low blood pressure, the patient is likely sleeping when drug concentrations are the highest. Encouraging patients who are on numerous blood pressure-lowering medications to get up slowly and be aware of dizziness and lightheadedness is important. Have an extra awareness of using alpha-blockers with other blood pressure-lowering medications in our geriatric population. Their baroreceptor reflex is not what it once was compared to a younger individual.

In addition to traditional antihypertensives, we must recognize the risk of hypotension when alpha-blockers are used in combination with other blood pressure-lowering medications. PDE-5 inhibitors like sildenafil and antipsychotics are both well known to contribute to orthostasis. There are countless other examples of medications that can have a blood pressure-lowering effect. Monitoring of blood pressure and patient awareness is critical.

Combining Tamsulosin and a Non-Selective Alpha-Blocker

Tamsulosin is more selective for bladder receptors than a non-selective agent like terazosin or doxazosin. This is a dose-dependent effect, so as we increase the tamsulosin dose, we may see that selectivity disappear. If the selectivity disappears, we will run into alpha-blocking activity on the vessels and a drop in blood pressure is likely.

I wanted to specifically mention the combination of Tamsulosin with a non-selective alpha-blocker because I have seen it numerous times in clinic practice. The most common situation that this happens is when the primary provider is not communicating appropriately with a specialty provider. Tamsulosin is never used for its blood pressure-lowering effect. The non-selective agents can be used for both blood pressure lowering effects and BPH. Because of this, you may see a patient with resistant hypertension put on a non-selective alpha-blocker. If the patient then develops BPH or other urinary symptoms that necessitate an alpha-blocker, tamsulosin will typically be used while ignoring or missing the fact that they are already taking an alpha-blocker for hypertension. Be aware of this potential duplication and the interaction that can result as there is an additive alpha-blocking effect that can cause serious hypotension. This combination should not be used together.

CYP3A4 Inhibition

Tamsulosin is contraindicated with the use of strong CYP3A4 inhibitors. Classic examples include itraconazole, systemic ketoconazole, clarithromycin and some of the HIV medications like cobicistat, lopinavir, and ritonavir. The result of this interaction is an elevation in the concentration of tamsulosin. Other drugs that inhibit CYP3A4 to a lesser degree are going to have varying impacts on the concentration of tamsulosin. Dosing of the CYP3A4 inhibitor, as well as tamsulosin, will have bearing on how significant the interaction is. The most likely complication from this would be a drop in blood pressure and risk for dizziness and falls.

Terazosin does avoid the CYP3A4 pathway. This could be a potential alternative if there is a desire for the use of a non-selective agent. Doxazosin does not. Being aware of these inter-class differences can be the difference between encountering side effects or not depending upon the other medications that your patient may be taking.

3A4 Inducers

Tamsulosin and doxazosin will both be affected negatively by CYP3A4 inducers. Concentrations of tamsulosin and doxazosin will go down when an inducer like phenytoin, rifampin, or carbamazepine is initiated. Recognize this risk in patients who may be reporting worsening symptoms of BPH or increases in blood pressure.

5-Alpha Reductase Inhibitors

Additive Effects

Saw palmetto is a supplement that is commonly taken by patients who have BPH. Saw palmetto has the potential to have similar effects to the 5-alpha reductase inhibitors. It would be reasonable to discontinue saw palmetto if the patient has significant enough symptoms to be placed on a 5-alpha-reductase inhibitor like finasteride or dutasteride. While the likelihood of complications from using these together is low, the theory is that it will have added antiandrogen type effects. In patients who are taking this combination, the risk for reduced testosterone effects would be possible. Keep an eye out for added effects like sexual dysfunction.

CYP3A4 Inhibition

Inhibitors of CYP3A4 could potentially have impacts on both dutasteride and finasteride. In general, the effects of this interaction could lead to mild increases in the concentration of each drug. While this is possible, it is unlikely that changes will need to be made because of alterations in the metabolic pathway.

Urinary Anticholinergics

Additive Effects

Urinary anticholinergics are frequently used to help manage incontinence symptoms. The urinary anticholinergics include medications like oxybutynin (Ditropan), tolterodine (Detrol), and solifenacin (Vesicare). They can help reduce the urge and frequency of urinary symptoms. Because urge incontinence and urinary frequency are typically more associated with the elderly, these drugs are more likely to be used in this patient population. Because of their anticholinergic nature, we are very likely to run into adverse effects. This can be complicated by the fact that many elderly may already be taking other anticholinergic medications.

Dry eyes, dry mouth, confusion, urinary retention, and constipation are all common complications from anticholinergic therapy. When urinary anticholinergics are combined with other drugs that have anticholinergic effects, we can potentiate the adverse effect profile. Watch out for combinations of diphenhydramine, hydroxyzine, TCAs, or any other agents that may have anticholinergic activity. Having awareness for medications that are managing these side effects is also critical.

Recognize that when patients require artificial tears, saliva supplements, dementia medications, or constipation medications, we may be having additive effects from the patient being on multiple anticholinergic medications.

Another term for this is "anticholinergic burden". The more medications that a patient takes with anticholinergic activity, the more likely that they will have anticholinergic type side effects.

In addition to the anticholinergic burden, we should also think about medications that have additive side effects regardless of the mechanism that causes those side effects. A great example of this is opioids. Opioids are going to cause constipation and when used in combination with anticholinergics, it can take constipation to another level requiring new constipation medications or increased dosages. Here's a different example where a medication like pseudoephedrine could have additive effects and opposing effects when combined with anticholinergics.

An 89 year old patient has been battling anxiety, symptoms of urinary retention, and insomnia over the previous few months. He has a history of GERD, hypertension, BPH, allergies with congestion, and constipation. Here's his medication list:
- lorazepam 0.25 mg twice daily as needed
- diphenhydramine 25 mg daily at bedtime
- omeprazole 20 mg daily
- lisinopril 20 mg daily
- metoprolol 25 mg twice daily
- hydrochlorothiazide 25 mg daily
- oxybutynin 10 mg daily
- pseudoephedrine 60 mg every 4-6 hours as needed
- clonidine 0.1 mg twice daily
- docusate 100 mg twice daily
- sennosides 2 tablets twice daily

The first thing I would look at addressing is the current problems mentioned above. With anxiety, insomnia, and urinary retention, I'd be concerned that the pseudoephedrine side effects are exacerbating these conditions and potentially causing unnecessary use of other medications. Timing is very important to assess when identifying drug reactions. It is only prescribed as needed, so we would need to assess if they are taking the pseudoephedrine, how often, and when did they start taking it? I'd also look and see if any of the blood pressure medications have been increased with the timing of the pseudoephedrine. We also have some issues with constipation. This is a perfect example of the potential of the prescribing cascade.

Is Sudafed (pseudoephedrine) worsening hypertension and therefore causing the use of more blood pressure medications? Is it causing insomnia necessitating the use of diphenhydramine? Is it causing or worsening anxiety and inciting the use of Ativan (lorazepam)? Is the diphenhydramine and oxybutynin in combination with the pseudoephedrine contributing to the adverse effect of urinary retention? Is the diphenhydramine contributing to constipation? These are a few important questions when assessing polypharmacy, drug interactions, and the prescribing cascade.

Opposing Effects

On the flip side of the spectrum, adding a urinary anticholinergic medication can directly oppose something else we may be trying to treat. A drug like oxybutynin can oppose the activity of acetylcholinesterase inhibitors like donepezil. This can lead to worsening cognition and memory problems.

The same principle applies to constipation medications or medications used to manage symptoms of BPH. Drugs with anticholinergic activity will directly oppose the benefit of medications to manage these conditions.

In patients with a diagnosis like gastroparesis, it is also important to recognize the effect of anticholinergic medications. These drugs slow down the gut and if we are using a medication like metoclopramide for gastroparesis, the anticholinergic medication will be in direct opposition to symptoms that we are trying to manage.

CYP3A4

Oxybutynin and tolterodine are probably the two agents I see used most often for symptoms of urinary frequency. These agents and their concentrations can be altered by changes in CYP3A4 metabolism. Much like other drugs, CYP3A4 inhibitors can raise concentrations while CYP3A4 inducers can lower concentrations. When an inhibitor is started, paying attention to the risk for anticholinergic side effects is important. If a 3A4 inducer is utilized, be aware that what was once an effective treatment may no longer be beneficial if the concentrations have been reduced to a significant extent.

CYP2D6

In addition to CYP3A4, tolterodine is also broken down by CYP2D6. Inhibitors of CYP2D6 would be likely to raise the concentrations of tolterodine and thus increasing the risk for anticholinergic adverse effects.

Lactic Acidosis Risk

Lactic acidosis is an extremely rare but serious adverse effect of metformin. If we think about the use of alcohol, even when it is used alone, it can increase the risk of lactic acidosis. The risk is generally more associated with binge type drinking, but using agents together that can both contribute to the risk should be recognized. To avoid the additive risk, it would be advisable to avoid the use of alcohol altogether. This may be undesirable for many patients and they may choose to drink alcohol anyway. If this is the case, it would be advisable to remind them of the risks and that the risk may be greater with excessive drinking.

There is also a significant risk for lactic acidosis when intravenous contrast media is used in a patient who takes metformin. This risk is due to the potential of contrast dye to cause acute renal failure. If this happens there is greater potential that metformin will accumulate and be more likely to cause lactic acidosis. Due to the risk of accumulation and lactic acidosis, metformin should be avoided in patients with substantial renal impairment. Typically, the metformin is held for 48 hours before and after the contrast.

OCT Inhibition

Organic cation transporters are an important way that drugs are eliminated in the body. The primary concern with these transporters in relation to metformin is their activity in the kidney. Metformin is a potential substrate of this transporter. Under normal conditions, metformin is transported (at least in part) into the urine through this transporter. This helps eliminate metformin from the body. There are drugs that can alter the function of OCTs in the kidneys. If this is the case, we can increase the concentrations of metformin and ultimately increase the likelihood of adverse effects and toxicity. Some medications that may impact this transporter include cimetidine, trimethoprim, dolutegravir, cephalosporins, and lamotrigine.

For many of these agents, we could select alternatives. If we do need to use a drug with OCT inhibition, monitoring for metformin toxicity and possibly reducing the dose would be appropriate. I would be even more concerned about this interaction if the patient already had preexisting renal issues.

Drugs That Increase Renal Failure Risk

Similar to IV contrast, we do have to recognize that any medication or medication combination that can cause acute renal failure can increase the risk of escalating metformin concentrations. With those elevations in metformin concentrations, we worry about the risk of lactic acidosis. Commonly used agents that may induce renal dysfunction or cause renal failure include diuretics, NSAIDs, ACE inhibitors, ARBs, aminoglycosides, and vancomycin.

Opposition of Beneficial Effects

Metformin is the first-line agent in the management of type 2 diabetes. We can have nice reductions in blood sugar and ultimately reduction in A1C. There are a few medications that can oppose the beneficial effects of metformin. The most common agent that can substantially raise blood sugars includes any systemic corticosteroid. Even injections can have meaningful effects on blood sugar. Other medications that can increase blood sugars and oppose the blood sugar lowering effects of metformin include antipsychotics (some more than others), thiazide diuretics, niacin, and drugs with stimulatory effects like pseudoephedrine.

Sulfonylureas

Increasing Risks of Hypoglycemia

Any medication that can lower blood sugar is going to increase the risk of hypoglycemia. Commonly used sulfonylureas include glipizide, glimepiride, and glyburide. Sulfonylureas directly stimulate the production and release of insulin. Because of this fact, they create an opportunity for hypoglycemia to happen. Pay attention to blood sugars when new medications are started or increased. Also, be sure that patients are aware of hypoglycemia and how to manage it.

In addition to virtually any medication used for type 2 diabetes, quinolone antibiotics have also been associated with altering blood sugars and potentially contributing to hypoglycemia. Quinolones aren't typically avoided due to this reason, but it would be a good education point particularly if the patient has struggled with hypoglycemia episodes in the past.

Masking Hypoglycemia

Beta-blockers are well known to blunt some of the signs and symptoms of hypoglycemia. When taking sulfonylureas or other medications that can cause hypoglycemia, we need to remember this. This is especially important in patients who are at risk for hypoglycemia.

It is even riskier if they have a past history of hypoglycemia, lower baseline blood sugars, or have cognitive impairment. It is something that should be considered, but beta-blockers are still often used in patients with diabetes and who may be taking a sulfonylurea. If hypoglycemia becomes a problem, we should be reassessing the use of sulfonylureas in favor of other agents that may not be as likely to cause hypoglycemia. It is also important to distinguish between cardioselective beta-blockers and non-selective beta-blockers. Non-selective beta-blockers like propranolol may be higher risk. Indication matters as well. If we are using a beta-blocker strictly for hypertension, we would likely consider another agent in its place. If we are using the beta-blocker for atrial fibrillation, there are other options for rate control, but if they were well controlled we would most likely look to alter the diabetes regimen.

CYP2C9 Inhibition

Many of the sulfonylureas are broken down by CYP2C9. Be able to recognize common CYP2C9 inhibitors as starting one can increase the likelihood of increased concentrations of a sulfonylurea and ultimately the possibility for hypoglycemia. Fluconazole is a common example of a drug that can inhibit CYP2C9. Being aware of baseline blood sugars is important in the situation of drug interactions. If a patient routinely has blood sugars in the 200's and above, I'm not going to be as likely to be concerned about hypoglycemia due to the interaction. If their fasting blood sugar is routinely 70-80, a small increase in the concentration of their sulfonylurea could easily lead to clinically significant and symptomatic hypoglycemia.

Appetite Changes and GI Upset

It is critical to recognize that many medications may alter appetite. On a short term basis, antibiotics are well known to cause nausea, diarrhea, and even vomiting in some cases. If this alteration in dietary intake occurs, patients who take sulfonylureas are going to be at risk of overstimulating the release of insulin for what they actually need. In situations like this, we are first going to encourage closer blood sugar monitoring. This is really our best defense against something bad happening in the short term. If it is an antibiotic or other agent causing significant adverse effects, we may look to change that medication. Depending upon the blood sugars, we may look to hold or reduce the dose of the sulfonylurea. If patients are experiencing hypoglycemia episodes and this has been a problem in the past as well, we might look to get away from the use of a sulfonylurea altogether and use some of the numerous other diabetes options.

SGLT-2 Inhibitors

Diuretic Effect

The SGLT-2 Inhibitors like empagliflozin, dapagliflozin, and canagliflozin are unique in how they help lower blood sugars. In general, they do not have many drug interactions. These drugs reduce blood sugar by increasing the output of blood glucose through the urine. In the transport of glucose out through the kidney and into the urine, water can also go with it. Because of this reduction in blood volume, there is a risk for volume depletion, dehydration, and lower blood pressure.

Adding an SGLT-2 to a diuretic may increase the likelihood of dizziness and low blood pressure. It also may increase the risk of acute renal failure through dehydration. Monitoring for dizziness and assessing blood pressure would be critical when considering adding an SGLT-2 to a patient already taking a diuretic. In addition, you would want to assess kidney function to ensure that the patient is not getting dehydrated.

SGLT-2 and Hypoglycemia

Hypoglycemia risk is low when these drugs are used as monotherapy in type 2 diabetes. You need to be more concerned about hypoglycemia when a patient is taking insulin or a drug that stimulates the release of insulin. Educating your patient to be aware of the signs and symptoms of hypoglycemia is critical. Checking blood sugars a little more frequently upon initiation would be another strategy to ensure that the patient isn't getting too low.

Hyperglycemia/Hypoglycemia

Much like the SGLT-2 inhibitors, the GLP-1 agonists like liraglutide, dulaglutide, and exenatide do not have a significant number of drug interactions which is a good thing. Be aware of other agents and current blood sugars when starting these agents. Patients who are started on drugs that can oppose the blood sugar lowering effect should be noted. Corticosteroids are by far the most commonly used drugs that can raise blood sugars. Extra monitoring should take place when these medications are used. Other agents like antipsychotics, estrogen, thiazide diuretics, tacrolimus, cyclosporine, and some HIV medications can also have varying degrees of effects. Keep in mind that the effect on blood sugar for these agents is typically going to be dose dependent. The higher the dose, the more likely it is that they will raise blood sugar. Much like any other blood sugar-lowering agents, the risk for hypoglycemia is significantly increased when the patient is taking insulin or sulfonylureas.

Slowing the Gut

It is important to remember how the GLP-1 agonists work. These drugs have action on the gut which slows it down and helps promote fullness. This is one reason why they can help with weight loss. However, this can be a negative if the gut is already at risk for being slowed down too much. Be aware of the potential additive effects of other gut slowing agents. Any medication with anticholinergic activity can slow down the GI tract and if added to a GLP-1 could have an added effect. Be aware of patients who may have gastroparesis or symptoms of gastroparesis.

Alcohol

Be aware that there have been case reports of pancreatitis with GLP-1's. This isn't very common, but it is important to think about patients who may be at risk for pancreatitis and consider other alternatives in those patients. In particular, if you have a patient with a known history of alcoholism, they will likely be at increased risk for pancreatitis. If you are deciding between a GLP-1 or another agent, this may be one factor that could steer you away from using a GLP-1.

Edema

Pioglitazone is well known to cause edema and weight gain. It is important to be aware of other medications that can have additive effects. NSAIDs are a common medication class that can cause sodium retention and increase the risk of edema. In addition, gabapentin, and pregabalin are well known to cause edema. Calcium channel blockers primarily used for hypertension can also contribute to edema. Recognize the additive risks of using pioglitazone with some of these medications. In patients with CHF, it is absolutely critical to avoid these combinations as we run the risk of causing exacerbations and fluid retention.

CYP2C8

We discussed the risk of gemfibrozil when used with pioglitazone earlier in the book. Pioglitazone concentrations can be increased in patients who are taking a CYP2C8 inhibitor like gemfibrozil. There are other drugs that can also inhibit CYP2C8 to varying degrees. Clopidogrel and trimethoprim are other examples of medications that can inhibit CYP2C8 and raise the concentrations of pioglitazone. This is an interaction that we are likely going to monitor. Lower blood sugars and a higher risk for adverse effects like edema would be the most likely outcomes from this interaction. With a drug like clopidogrel, we are unlikely to discontinue this agent because of this interaction. If adverse effects from the pioglitazone were encountered, we'd be more likely to change the pioglitazone. Pioglitazone seems to be falling out of favor due to its negative side effect profile of weight gain and edema in favor of agents like GLP-1 agonists and SGLT-2's.

Blood Sugar Alterations

Much like all of the other medications used in diabetes, recognizing agents that may oppose the blood sugar lowering effect and agents that may cause hypoglycemia is important. We should monitor blood sugars more closely when drugs are added or discontinued that are known to affect blood sugar.

Angioedema

DPP-4 inhibitors like sitagliptin and linagliptin have a pretty low risk for drug interactions. On the less common side of the drug interactions scale, there have been sparse reports of angioedema. Be aware of patients who have a past history of angioedema due to medications or those who may be on higher risk medications like ACE inhibitors, sacubitril/valsartan, or ARBs. In the overwhelming majority of situations, angioedema isn't likely to be a reason that you avoid using the medication, but you may want to do a little extra patient education and monitoring if you think they may be at risk.

Insulin

Hypoglycemia

The same principles that apply to sulfonylureas will apply to insulin. Insulin can cause hypoglycemia on its own, but the risk tends to rise as we add other antidiabetic agents to the patient's regimen. Be aware of risk factors for hypoglycemia, baseline sugars, dietary changes, cognition changes, and other factors that may affect the occurrence of hypoglycemia.

Hyperglycemia

In the same respect as other diabetes medications, recall that many agents can raise blood sugars to varying degrees. Recognize that the use of corticosteroids, certain immunosuppressives, and thiazides all may impact the blood sugar control of our patients who have been stabilized on insulin.

Heart Failure

In addition to the risk of hypoglycemia, there is another risk when combining insulin with pioglitazone. Patients who take this combination have been shown to have an increased risk for heart failure exacerbations. Avoidance of pioglitazone in the heart failure population is the best course of action. If you recall, pioglitazone is contraindicated in patients with New York Heart Association Class III or IV heart failure. Canadian labeling actually recommends avoiding pioglitazone in any stage of heart failure.

Masking Hypoglycemia

Beta-blockers are well known to blunt some of the signs and symptoms of hypoglycemia. One unique symptom of hypoglycemia is sweating. This symptom is typically unaffected by the use of beta-blockers. Educating patients that they may still experience sweating if they are having a hypoglycemic episode can be an important point of emphasis in those taking a beta-blocker. Avoiding non-selective agents like nadolol and propranolol is a solid recommendation.

Levothyroxine and Thyroid Products

Binding Interactions

Without a doubt, binding interactions are the most important concern when it comes to drug interactions and levothyroxine. When levothyroxine is in the gut, there are numerous drugs and supplements that can bind to it. This leads to a reduction in the percentage of levothyroxine that is absorbed in the gut. Because less levothyroxine is absorbed, we are likely going to precipitate hypothyroidism.

Examples of common medications and supplements that can bind up levothyroxine include magnesium, aluminum hydroxide, cholestyramine, calcium, iron, raloxifene, and ciprofloxacin.

Consistency is key to the use of levothyroxine. If a patient has been taking levothyroxine with another agent that it can interact with but their TSH has been fine and the patient is asymptomatic, we are likely going to leave it alone and recommend that the patient continues to take the levothyroxine the way they have always been taking it.

Levothyroxine use is typically chronic. When we add new medications, we need to think about the timing of these medications. Separation is an acceptable way to handle these binding interactions. The nice thing about levothyroxine is that it is only dosed once daily. Because of this, we can dose it early in the morning and then take any other medications that may interact with it later in the day.

If there is doubt about a patient being affected by a binding interaction, we have an alternative to dealing with this. We can always check a TSH 6-8 weeks after initiating a new medication that we think may affect the absorption of levothyroxine. This can help ensure that the patient is remaining euthyroid.

Opposition Of Levothyroxine

There are agents that can impact levothyroxine concentrations beyond affecting absorption. Carbamazepine has the potential to induce the metabolism of levothyroxine. This can result in low concentrations of thyroid hormone. If carbamazepine is started, it would be advisable to check levels and monitor for patient symptoms. Amiodarone, estrogen, phenytoin, and rifampin are other examples of medications that can impact thyroid function. We need to be checking levels and assessing for symptoms of hypothyroidism in these patients when these medications are started or doses are changed.

Testosterone

Cyclosporine

Testosterone has the potential to raise cyclosporine concentrations. Because of this, we need to be extremely careful in a transplant patient. The tight therapeutic index of cyclosporine makes it necessary to monitor cyclosporine concentrations and recognize signs and symptoms of cyclosporine toxicity. GI adverse effects can result from acute toxicity. Liver failure, elevations in potassium, and immunosuppression are also risks associated with elevated cyclosporine concentrations.

Warfarin

Increased warfarin concentrations have been reported when it is used in combination with testosterone. Checking INR more closely and assessing for bleeding signs and symptoms is critical to managing this drug interaction.

Hypoglycemia Risk

In patients with diabetes, it is important to note that androgens like testosterone can increase the risk of hypoglycemia. Monitoring blood sugar following initiation would be important in any patient taking medication for type 2 diabetes. I would recommend placing more emphasis on monitoring for patients who have a history of hypoglycemia and are taking insulin or sulfonylureas.

Edema

Edema is a potential adverse effect of testosterone products. Pay attention to patients who may be on other medications that may increase this risk. Pioglitazone, corticosteroids, pregabalin, gabapentin, and calcium channel blockers are common examples of medication that could increase fluid retention and symptoms of edema.

CYP2C19 Inhibition

The citalopram and omeprazole interaction is a challenging one. As a clinical pharmacist, I don't want to create a bunch of other work or switch agents when medication therapy is working and justified. I feel like we (MDs, NPs, and PAs as well) often get put in this situation where there is an interaction that can cause really serious problems, but the risk for that outcome is extremely rare.

So how can citalopram be affected by omeprazole? With this interaction, the concentration of citalopram can be increased due to the inhibition of CYP2C19 by omeprazole. Higher concentrations of citalopram could lead to potential adverse effects. Serotonin syndrome and QTc prolongation are two very rare, but obviously serious adverse effects that could happen with this interaction. When you have increased concentrations of citalopram, you run the risk of prolonging the QT interval. Again, the risk of something serious like Torsades de Pointes is extremely rare. Here's what I would consider.

Look at the doses of each agent. If they are both low doses, this likely isn't a big deal.

I would also recommend reviewing the latest EKG. If the QTc value is solid within the normal range and they have been on citalopram and omeprazole (or esomeprazole) at the time the EKG was taken, there's no reason to be highly concerned.

Look at the other medications. If other medications are on the list that can prolong the QT interval, I may be a little more concerned. Antipsychotics, antiemetics, and some antiarrhythmics are a few examples. Looking at risk factors like electrolyte imbalances in magnesium and potassium is also important.

If I felt that something needed to be done with this interaction, here's what I would consider changing. Changing the PPI to an H2 blocker would potentially be a pretty easy switch. That is probably where I would start. There may be situations where that isn't possible.

In addition to changing to another class of medication, we could also look for an individual PPI that may affect CYP2C19 to a lesser extent or not at all. Pantoprazole would be less likely to raise concentrations of citalopram. Changing to esomeprazole would not be helpful as it interacts with citalopram as well.

Depending upon the depression symptoms and effectiveness of citalopram, you could consider changing the SSRI. Sertraline would not have this interaction as it avoids CYP2C19 metabolism.

Another option to consider is to do an EKG. If there isn't a recent one on record and you are concerned, this is certainly a viable option.

I would say in the majority of situations, I'm probably going to leave this drug interaction alone. Many times, a chronic PPI isn't necessary, so that is a great way to tackle polypharmacy and avoid the interaction. This can be challenging, however, especially if you work in a setting where access to clinical information is limited.

Clopidogrel, escitalopram, and tacrolimus are examples of three other medications that may be impacted by CYP2C19 inhibition. The clinical activity of clopidogrel would likely be reduced by this interaction, but escitalopram and tacrolimus concentrations would likely be increased. The clopidogrel omeprazole interaction was discussed further in the cardiovascular section.

Acid Suppression – Drug Absorption

PPIs are used to reduce the production of gastric acid. Commonly used PPIs include omeprazole, pantoprazole, lansoprazole, rabeprazole, esomeprazole, and dexlansoprazole. These drugs can be of great help in managing symptoms of ulcers and heartburn, but they can lead to some potentially negative consequences. There are some medications that are better absorbed in a low pH (or acidic) environment. We discussed iron supplementation under the supplement section. Oral iron is much better absorbed under acidic conditions. Another medication that can have absorption significantly altered is oral cefuroxime. Cefuroxime is a cephalosporin antibiotic used to treat certain bacterial infections. Another less common, but rare interaction is with erlotinib. Erlotinib is indicated for certain types of lung and pancreatic cancers. Lower bioavailability and reduced concentrations in the blood could be very serious for a patient who is using the medication to treat cancer. One last example to demonstrate this concept is atazanavir. Atazanavir can be used as part of an antiretroviral regimen for the management of HIV. This drug is poorly absorbed in a high pH environment that PPIs create.

Enzyme Inducers

Drugs like rifampin and St. John's Wort can induce CYP2C19 and other CYP enzymes as well. This can reduce the concentrations of many of the PPIs. Be aware of patients who have a return in heartburn or ulcer symptoms. It may be due to this interaction causing subtherapeutic concentrations. We likely have no solid medical purpose for St. John's Wort, so discontinuing this would likely be my primary solution. In the event of using rifampin, we could look for other antibiotic options or reassess how critical the PPI is to the patient's medication regimen.

B12 Deficiency

PPIs are associated with B12 deficiency. This means that they could potentially counteract the effects of B12 supplementation. In addition to blunting the effects of supplementation, there could be additive effects of B12 deficiency in patients who are taking metformin in combination with a PPI. Also, recall that patients with alcoholism are at risk for numerous nutritional deficiencies. B12 can be one of these and PPIs may further contribute to this issue. Assessing B12 levels periodically could be considered as well as monitoring and identifying symptoms of deficiency like anemia, neuropathy, and cognitive impairment.

Opposing Effects

As part of the long term side effect profile, PPIs can contribute to osteoporosis risk. In patients who are being treated for osteoporosis with drugs like alendronate or denosumab, PPI adverse effects can oppose the benefits of these medications. When PPIs are being used long term, be sure that the dose is minimized and that a periodic reassessment of benefit is done. Barrett's esophagus or chronic peptic ulcers are two examples of indications where long term PPI use will likely be appropriate and there may not be much we can do. Long term use of PPIs after stress ulcer prophylaxis in the hospital or added due to stomach upset are examples where we should not use PPIs long term.

Cimetidine

Cimetidine needs to be mentioned in its own special category amongst the H2 blockers. The reason it gets specifically mentioned is that it can inhibit numerous CYP enzymes and have very clinically significant impacts like the case below.

An 85 year old female with an extensive seizure history is taking phenytoin 300 mg daily. The previous phenytoin level was 14 and the patient was not displaying any signs or symptoms of toxicity. She began having some GI complaints and was diagnosed with GERD and put on cimetidine. About 2 weeks later, it was noted that the nurses had described the resident as having a decline in status, increased confusion, difficulty walking, and increased sedation. A Dilantin level was eventually ordered. For those of you not familiar with general target concentrations of phenytoin levels, the usual standard is about 10-20 micrograms/mL with some exceptions. Alterations in albumin can make this value not completely accurate and there is an equation to correct for this. In any case, this patient's total phenytoin level came back at 33! The team taking care of this patient was very fortunate that it was caught in time, avoiding hospitalization or worse! Cimetidine has a lot of substantial drug interactions and if you ever see it utilized, be sure you're thinking about this.

Cimetidine can inhibit CYP3A4 which as you should know by now can wreak havoc on many medications. Concentrations of drugs like amiodarone, diltiazem, phenytoin, and warfarin can all be substantially altered in an upward direction. As you can see from the case above, by inhibiting CYP3A4 drug toxicity can result. One of the great mysteries of the Food and Drug Administration (the agency in charge of determining whether a medication is over-the-counter or prescription only) is that cimetidine, with all of its drug interactions, still remains classified as an over-the-counter medication. Any patient can go purchase this medication without a healthcare provider's prescription or consent.

In addition to CYP3A4 inhibition, cimetidine can also have action on CYP2D6 and CYP1A2. Concentrations of paroxetine may go up if a patient is taking a CYP2D6 inhibitor. Concentrations of a drug like tizanidine may rise if cimetidine is started due to the CYP1A2 inhibition. If an H2 blocker is being selected, cimetidine should be avoided due to numerous potential drug interactions.

Acid Suppression – Drug Absorption

With the exception of cimetidine as mentioned above, H2 blockers as a class generally aren't considered to have a lot of drug interactions and most of them would be associated with their potential to alter the pH of the stomach.

Much like the PPIs, when H2 blockers like ranitidine or famotidine are utilized, our intent is to reduce stomach acid. By reducing acid production, we can help relieve symptoms of heartburn and GI ulceration, but drugs that may require a lower pH for absorption can be affected.

All of the examples discussed in the PPI section would apply here. Iron and cefuroxime are two of the more common examples that may be affected. It is very important to remember that this is going to only be oral formulations. By using IV formulations of drugs, we bypass the gut and absorption through the GI tract.

With cefuroxime, we can try to alter the timing of administration which may modestly help. At least a couple of hours of separation would be mandatory to help improve the absorption of the cefuroxime. With so many other cephalosporines available, my best solution would be to look toward a different antibiotic.

In managing the oral iron supplement interaction, separation of the drug administration time may be a prudent step. I have seen situations where they have been given together and the iron level did respond. I wouldn't recommend giving them at the same time. Lab monitoring and clinical response to iron are critical to watch for. The most common reason a patient would take iron is for iron deficiency anemia. By checking a CBC, we can assess hemoglobin and make sure that it is responding to iron replacement. In addition, we can check ferritin to assess iron stores and make sure the iron is being absorbed.

OCT2 Inhibition

There is some evidence that H2 blockers may have varying degrees of OCT2 inhibition. Because of this, certain drug concentrations may be mildly impacted. Varenicline, used for smoking cessation, is an example of a medication that may have its concentrations increased due to this potential interaction. Be aware of the adverse effect profile of varenicline which would have you looking for side effects like CNS changes, abnormal dreams, and GI upset.

QTc Prolongation

There are three significant concerns that I think of when I see a prescription for ondansetron. The first one is the risk for QTc prolongation. In the overwhelming majority of patients, I won't have a high level of concern. However, if I see that a patient is taking other agents that can have additive effects when it comes to QTc prolongation, I stop and reassess.

Common agents (not an all-inclusive list) that you have to be aware of as far as the risk of QTc prolongation include amiodarone and other antiarrhythmics, quinolone antibiotics, macrolide antibiotics, TCAs, certain SSRIs (most commonly citalopram and escitalopram) and antipsychotics. In addition to drug risk factors, there are other clinical findings that may alter your risk calculation. Assessing a baseline QTc value is important. The level of concern may start to get a little higher as you rise above 450ms or higher. Concern should be very high in patients who have a baseline QTc of 500ms. Other risk factors may include preexisting heart damage from heart failure, MI, or valvular disease. In addition, recognize that lower levels of potassium and magnesium may also place a patient at higher risk for the life-threatening situation of Torsades de pointes.

Serotonin Syndrome

Ondansetron has been associated with serotonin syndrome in patients taking other serotonergic drugs. Serotonin syndrome is extremely rare, but in a patient who is beginning to take ondansetron, it would be a good idea to take a quick review of their medication list to assess if and how many serotonergic medications they are taking. The most common agents that are going to raise the risk for serotonin syndrome include SSRIs, TCAs, SNRIs, tramadol, and MAOIs.

In addition to recognizing which drugs have serotonergic activity, I would pay attention to doses. A patient taking unusually high doses of one of these medications is more likely to precipitate serotonin syndrome than a patient who is taking small doses. Comparing a patient who is taking fluoxetine 10 mg compared to a patient taking sertraline 300 mg is a no-brainer as far as serotonin syndrome risk. Adding ondansetron to the patient taking sertraline 300 mg is going to have a higher risk of creating serotonin syndrome versus the patient taking low dose fluoxetine.

In addition to the dose, think about the number of medications that have serotonergic activity. If you have a patient who is taking a TCA like amitriptyline for migraines, citalopram for depression, tramadol for pain and we add in a PRN dose of ondansetron, we are putting that patient at greater risk for serotonin syndrome to occur.

With serotonin syndrome being extremely rare, you likely won't run into this, but if your patient has a past history of serotonin syndrome, we need to be even more careful with serotonergic drugs and combinations of agents that may increase serotonin activity.

Most importantly, if you do have concerns for serotonin syndrome risk, educating your patient about the risk is important so they are not hesitant about seeking appropriate medical attention if necessary.

Opposition of Beneficial Effects

The last interaction I want to mention with ondansetron is the potential to use medications that can have opposing effects. With its ability to relieve nausea and vomiting symptoms, we have numerous medications that can cause those problems with their adverse effect profile. Recognize drugs that may have been started prior to starting ondansetron. GLP-1 agonists, carbidopa/levodopa, metformin, antibiotics, chemotherapy, NSAIDs, and colchicine are all common agents that may cause nausea and precipitate the use of ondansetron if those adverse effects go unrecognized. In the case of chemotherapy and possibly other treatments, the benefits of treatment will likely outweigh the risks of nausea and vomiting. In that situation, it is acceptable to use a medication to manage the opposing side effects of another medication.

Docusate

Mineral Oil and Docusate

Docusate is likely not going to be a problem because of its risk for drug interaction. The one exception is mineral oil. The likelihood that a patient is using both of these medications is extremely low, but they are both over-the-counter, so the potential for patient access is there.

Docusate has the potential to increase the systemic absorption of mineral oil. Mineral oil can accumulate in certain tissue like the liver and cause damage. Because of this and the fact that mineral oil can cause lung damage when aspirated, it is best to avoid mineral oil altogether as a management strategy for constipation.

Polyethylene Glycol

Digoxin

Polyethylene glycol (Miralax) for constipation has very minimal drug interactions. One potential interaction is digoxin. There is a concern that digoxin concentrations may be modestly reduced when used in combination with polyethylene glycol. Given the fact that polyethylene glycol is often only given on an as-needed basis, a periodic dose of this would be unlikely to result in any serious negative effects. If a patient is taking it daily, we could anticipate the risk of lowering digoxin concentrations would be a little higher. With that stated, if both are absolutely necessary, altering the timing of these doses could be helpful in avoiding this drug interaction. I'd recommend taking one of them at night and the other in the morning.

Promethazine

Dopamine Antagonist

By remembering the mechanism of action of individual drugs, we can anticipate how and why they are going to interact with other medications. Promethazine has dopamine blocking activity. With this activity, we need to think about medications that may oppose or add to this effect.

Be aware of patients who are taking dopamine agonists or dopamine replacement with carbidopa/levodopa. Promethazine can directly oppose the benefits of these medications. Carbidopa/levodopa can be particularly concerning in that patients may have an exacerbation of troublesome Parkinson's symptoms when promethazine is started.

Antipsychotics and other nausea agents like metoclopramide have dopamine blocking activity. By adding promethazine to a patient already taking an antipsychotic or metoclopramide, we run the risk of inducing movement disorder adverse effects. These combinations should generally be avoided and other agents like ondansetron should be considered in place of promethazine if we are managing nausea and vomiting symptoms.

Anticholinergic Activity

While not incredibly strong like diphenhydramine, promethazine has anticholinergic activity. Assessing the risk of other agents the patient may be taking that can add to the anticholinergic burden is important. Also be sure to assess patients for sneaky side effects like dry mouth, dry eyes, urinary retention, and constipation. In my experience, patients don't seem to report these side effects very often because they simply find them a nuisance or consider them normal with the aging process. But when asked, they often recognize that they have been having more trouble with them since starting a new anticholinergic agent.

Sedation

Promethazine is sedating. Recognize that this medication may need to be addressed if the patient is experiencing significant somnolence and taking other medications that may have additive sedation side effects.

Dicyclomine

Anticholinergic Burden

Dicyclomine is most frequently used for its antispasmodic activity in the GI tract. It can help manage symptoms of diarrhea and GI spasms most often associated with irritable bowel syndrome. It is a highly anticholinergic medication. Like with other anticholinergics, we need to be aware of the adverse effect profile and how it might affect other medications and disease states.

Urinary retention, dry eyes, dry mouth, constipation, sedation, and confusion are all potential risks associated with the use of dicyclomine. Be aware of patients who are taking medications for BPH. Dicyclomine's effects will directly oppose the beneficial effects of medications like alpha-blockers. Dicyclomine can also oppose any benefit from dementia medications.

Remembering the way anticholinergics can slow down the gut is important. Because of this, recall that the drug interaction with oral potassium tablets will occur with dicyclomine just like it can with any other anticholinergic medication. The opposition of prokinetic agents like metoclopramide or erythromycin can also be a problem associated with the use of dicyclomine. The gut slowing effects can be exacerbated by the use of opioids. An increased risk for constipation is a concern with using an anticholinergic and an opioid. Additive effects of dry mouth can also occur when using respiratory anticholinergics.

Fluticasone (Nasal)

CYP3A4 Inhibition

When I think about nasal steroids, significant risk for HPA suppression doesn't come to mind as systemic bioavailability is very low at <2%. However, there are some recommendations to avoid potent CYP3A4 inhibitors. CYP3A4 inhibitors are likely to prolong the half-life of fluticasone and may lead to an increased risk of systemic steroid exposure. While strong 3A4 inhibitors aren't used routinely in clinical practice, there are some drugs that you may see. Medications I've seen used in practice include ritonavir, lopinavir, itraconazole, ketoconazole, posaconazole, voriconazole, and clarithromycin. Because many of these agents aren't used long term, particularly the anti-infectives, this interaction isn't likely to cause adrenal suppression because the anti-infective will be discontinued relatively quickly.

With nasal fluticasone, I would also want to inquire about the patient's use. Even though this medication is often scheduled, some patients will only use it on an as-needed basis. Patients will often use it as needed throughout the year and may take it routinely during their difficult seasonal allergies (sometimes up to a month or two). If they are not taking it on a regular basis, the CYP3A4 inhibition interaction is going to be even less significant.

Montelukast

CYP2C8 Inhibition

Montelukast is pretty clean when it comes to drug interactions. CYP2C8 may play a role in helping breakdown this medication, so any drug that inhibits this enzyme has the potential to raise concentrations of montelukast. Gemfibrozil is an example of a medication that can inhibit CYP2C8. If they have to be used together, keep an eye out for signs of montelukast adverse effects. Typically montelukast is pretty well tolerated. Rarely I have seen some central nervous system changes from montelukast toxicity such as dizziness and fatigue. You may also rarely encounter GI adverse effects. There have been some case reports of psychiatric changes such as agitation, depression, and anxiety.

To address this interaction, most of the time we would likely be able to use fenofibrate in place of the gemfibrozil. Recall that gemfibrozil is more likely to have other significant drug interactions compared to fenofibrate, so this is another potential purpose to avoid its use.

Beta-Blockers

Recall that montelukast can be used in the management of allergies as well as asthma symptoms. If a patient is taking montelukast for asthma and experiencing worsening symptoms of asthma, remember to check for the use of beta-blockers which could exacerbate breathing and oppose the beneficial effects from montelukast.

Loratadine and Second Generation Antihistamines

Anticholinergic Activity

Loratadine is classified as having anticholinergic activity. All of the previous anticholinergic effects that we talked about in previous sections apply here. However, the extent to which they apply is much lower. Loratadine is much less anticholinergic than the first-generation antihistamines like hydroxyzine and diphenhydramine. Within the prescribing information of tiotropium, it actually lists that loratadine should not be used in combination due to the additive anticholinergic potential. When used at standard, therapeutic doses, the likelihood of loratadine and tiotropium causing more problems than dry mouth is pretty low. It is important to recognize other medications that may have anticholinergic activity and recognize that there can be a cumulative effect from patients who take combinations of multiple anticholinergic drugs. The fewer number of drugs with anticholinergic activity we can use, the better. This is especially true if a patient is experiencing adverse effects like urinary retention, confusion, tachycardia, dry eyes, dry mouth, and constipation.

On occasion, I have seen combinations of first-generation antihistamines like diphenhydramine and second-generation antihistamines like loratadine used together. This is not a combination I would recommend and the primary reason is the increased risk for anticholinergic side effects. Here's a case scenario demonstrating anticholinergic burden and how to approach medications.

An elderly patient was on Zyrtec (cetirizine) 10 mg at bedtime for allergies, diphenhydramine 25 mg for sleep, and was also on Ditropan (oxybutynin) 15 mg three times daily for urinary incontinence. Ditropan is one of those classic older anticholinergic medications that isn't so great in the elderly (noted to be in the Beer's criteria). This patient was experiencing significant dry mouth and dry eyes likely due to a heavy anticholinergic burden. The physician was concerned with the Zyrtec causing the anticholinergic symptoms because that was the most recent medication started. The diphenhydramine and oxybutynin were overlooked.

Patients will often self-treat and take over-the-counter medications like diphenhydramine. If a thorough review of the medication list is not done, this will often be missed. I was taught a couple of ways to remember a few of the major anticholinergic effects. Some use the acronym SLUDs – Meaning you CANNOT salivate, lacrimate, urinate, or defecate. Others use the saying "you can't spit, see, pee or poop" to describe anticholinergic effects. If you like to make things rhyme, you can substitute your curse word for poop. CNS effects like confusion, dizziness, and fall risk are also problematic with anticholinergic medications in the elderly.

Keeping an eye out for "trigger" medications that treat these symptoms is really important. Examples include artificial tears or saliva for dry eyes or dry mouth, respectively. Alpha-blockers like Flomax due to retention and donepezil for dementia symptoms are also medications that you may see added following the initiation of an anticholinergic medication.

In this case, if incontinence was well controlled, the Ditropan would likely be the medication I would be strongly advocating to decrease as 45 mg total daily dose is a very steep dose compared to the anticholinergic activity that 10 mg of Zyrtec would have. After reviewing the history of the Ditropan, I would assess and hopefully find an alternative to the diphenhydramine.

QTc Prolongation

I wouldn't immediately think of QTc prolongation when I think about second-generation antihistamines, but we can put it on the radar. This is especially true if a patient is taking amiodarone. In addition to the QTc prolonging nature of amiodarone, it can inhibit CYP3A4 which may increase the concentrations of loratadine and exacerbate its QTc prolonging risk. If a patient has seasonal allergies and hasn't tried anything yet, shifting a patient to a nasal corticosteroid might be an appropriate step. If it is desired to continue with the loratadine, we can monitor the EKG to ensure that we don't have a preexisting problem and that we aren't worsening it.

Cetirizine does avoid the CYP3A4 pathway more than loratadine and might be considered as an alternative in a patient taking amiodarone.

Sedation

Pretty much any antihistamine medication is going to have sedative properties. The second-generation antihistamines were developed to help reduce the risk of sedation. There are patient populations that should be monitored a little more closely. Be aware of patients who are taking other sedatives as we may have a cumulative type effect. Drugs like opioids, skeletal muscle relaxants, benzodiazepines, sleepers, and some antidepressants are a few examples of medications that may have additive sedative properties.

In comparing loratadine and cetirizine, cetirizine is typically considered a little more sedating than loratadine. In patients on multiple sedating agents, trying loratadine first might be considered. Responses to antihistamines can be variable. Because of this, we often employ a trial and error strategy as to which antihistamine is going to work better for a specific patient.

Diphenhydramine and the First Generation Antihistamines

Anticholinergic Activity

Diphenhydramine is a black sheep in the world of geriatrics. No one wants to use it if possible because it is highly anticholinergic. Hydroxyzine is another commonly used first-generation antihistamine that will have similar properties. To avoid the high anticholinergic burden of these agents, the second-generation agents like loratadine are typically preferred.

This does depend on the indication. Occasionally you will see hydroxyzine or diphenhydramine used for its sedative and anti-anxiety properties. If sedation or anxiety relief is the clinical desire, they will likely be more effective than second-generation agents. This does not remove the fact that you are much more likely to encounter anticholinergic adverse effects. Assessing the anticholinergic burden is critical in patients who we are going to use these medications.

Limiting the frequency of use and attempting to make these agents as needed only can hopefully help minimize their use and reduce the potential for anticholinergic adverse effects. In addition to an unusual dose of Flomax, here's a medication list where anticholinergic effects likely contributed to problems with BPH.

- Proscar 5 mg daily
- Nortriptyline 50 mg at bedtime
- Hydrochlorothiazide 12.5 mg daily
- Prednisone 10 mg daily
- Nexium 20 mg daily
- Flomax 0.8 mg twice daily
- Imdur 30 mg daily
- Aspirin 325 mg daily
- Metoprolol 25 mg twice daily
- Pseudoephedrine as needed
- Diphenhydramine 50 mg daily as needed for sleep
- Metformin 500 mg twice daily

BPH with urinary retention can be exacerbated by anticholinergic medications and there are two medications that I would look at first, with the exception of the Flomax dose.

I would want to know this patient's blood pressure and assess the Flomax dose first. If this dose is correct, I would be very nervous about this and addressing this with the patient and/or provider would be my top priority.

Anticholinergics can exacerbate BPH. In this case, you must figure out if this patient is using the diphenhydramine. Diphenhydramine in combination with the nortriptyline can substantially increase the anticholinergic burden.

Pseudoephedrine can contribute to both BPH and hypertension. Assessing for dosing as well as the frequency of as needed use would be very important.

Sedation

Even more so than the second-generation agents, first-generation antihistamines are very sedating. This is a dose-dependent effect so higher doses are more concerning than lower doses. In addition, this can be an additive effect when patients are taking other sedating medications. Assessing the indication and appropriateness of each sedating medication is critical. In addition, since sedative effects are generally tied to higher doses, we should look at each sedative medication to ensure that we are at the minimum effective dose.

126

It is important to note that there is a topical formulation of diphenhydramine. In the case of small areas of itching, this would be a potential option to help relieve symptoms at a low risk of systemic toxicity. Diphenhydramine can be absorbed to an extent through the skin so I would not recommend a bath in diphenhydramine cream, but this would be an option for small areas on the skin to likely avoid sedation as well as systemic anticholinergic effects.

Liver Toxicity

While acetaminophen has a pretty short list of drug interactions, it is well known to cause liver toxicity especially in combination with certain medications and at excessively high doses. Liver toxicity with acetaminophen is rare when patients are taking it at or under 4,000 mg per day. There are certain medications that can increase the risk of liver toxicity. Drugs like carbamazepine, isoniazid, and phenytoin can all contribute to liver issues alone, but when used in combination with acetaminophen, this risk may be higher.

The first thing I would consider when looking at these interactions is to assess if acetaminophen is necessary on a routine basis. If we can get by with as-needed use, we should try to do that. Alternatively, I would look to an alternative medicine for pain management. NSAIDs aren't ideal and will likely have plenty of drug and disease interactions to monitor, but maybe a consideration in a patient at risk for liver toxicity. Changing the other agents can be considered, but maybe less of an option than changing the acetaminophen.

Limiting the dose of acetaminophen is also a strategy that I have seen employed in an attempt to reduce liver toxicity risk. Lowering the maximum recommended dose for a patient who is on these medications to 3,000 mg or 2,000 mg per day is a consideration.

Monitoring liver function is going to be important. Patients who have risk factors for liver dysfunction are of significant concern. Pay attention if your patient uses alcohol or has a history of alcoholism. These patients can be at very high risk for liver problems and using multiple medications that can contribute to liver toxicity can be very dangerous.

Warfarin

Warfarin can interact with acetaminophen. I wouldn't call this a very strong drug interaction but it should be one that you are aware of. We typically don't change acetaminophen to something like an NSAID because NSAIDs are way riskier with anticoagulation than acetaminophen. Instead, we will typically just monitor the INR and adjust the dose of warfarin accordingly. Also, keep in mind that there is a dose-dependent difference in this interaction. If a patient is taking acetaminophen consistently once per day for the last year and the INR is at goal, this interaction has been accounted for.

If the acetaminophen is new and the patient goes from not taking acetaminophen to taking 2-4 grams per day, then an elevation in the INR at the next check will be much more likely. Bottom line is that acetaminophen is an acceptable choice in a patient on warfarin, but we should monitor the INR if patients are changing how much and how often they are taking it.

Vaccines

One unique interaction with acetaminophen is its potential to blunt the effectiveness of vaccines. Years ago, it was common practice to give acetaminophen with vaccines to prophylactically manage pain and fever that may be associated. However, there is some data that may indicate the immune response to vaccines may be blunted. Because of this, it would be best to avoid the use of acetaminophen for the management of mild to moderate pain or fever associated with a vaccine.

NSAIDs

There are numerous NSAIDs that are used in clinical practice. Some of the more common agents include ibuprofen (Motrin, Advil), meloxicam (Mobic), naproxen (Naprosyn, Aleve), and diclofenac (Voltaren). I will also include the COX-2 inhibitor celecoxib (Celebrex) in this group as many of the drug interactions are similar. The one primary advantage of celecoxib may be a lower risk of GI bleed.

Acute Kidney Injury

NSAIDs work on the afferent arteriole. The afferent arteriole is the vessel running into the glomerulus of the kidney. NSAIDs through their actions on prostaglandins can cause vasoconstriction on the afferent arteriole. This essentially allows less fluid to come into the glomerulus and effectively reduces the overall pressure. This loss in pressure to the glomerulus can inhibit the function and lead to AKI.

I discussed this in more depth when I talked about ACE inhibitors, ARBs, and diuretics. This combination of drugs can significantly raise the risk of acute renal failure. Close monitoring for elevations in creatinine from baseline is one of the most important ways to monitor this interaction. Particular attention should be given when these drugs are started or increased. In addition, patients who may be at risk for dehydration may have an even higher risk for acute renal failure.

CHF – Opposition of Diuresis

NSAIDs can reduce the production of prostaglandins that help the kidney function normally. A critical function of the kidney is to maintain salt and water homeostasis. Because NSAIDs can upset the prostaglandin supply, they can ultimately cause fluid retention and directly oppose the benefit that diuretics may be providing in heart failure. Here's a case scenario where adding an NSAID led to a worsening of heart failure symptoms requiring escalating doses of furosemide.

An 88 year old male has a history of osteoarthritis. He has tried self-treatment with acetaminophen 325 mg twice daily with no benefit. Upon a recent evaluation with his primary provider, he was prescribed naproxen 500 mg two times daily.

His current medication list includes:
- Lasix 20 mg daily
- Enalapril 10 mg daily
- Amlodipine 2.5 mg daily
- Metoprolol 12.5 mg twice daily
- Aspirin 325 mg daily
- Sucralfate 1 gm four times daily
- Senna S 2 tablets daily

Within a few weeks following the addition of naproxen 500 mg twice daily, our patient began to experience worsening shortness of breath, an increase of swelling in his ankles, and his weight increased by 6 pounds. He was diagnosed with a CHF exacerbation. Lasix was increased from 20 to 40 mg daily to help manage the situation. The NSAID likely contributed to the exacerbation.

Playing hindsight, this is a case where you would strongly try to avoid NSAIDs. It is always critical to assess if patients have had an adequate trial of a medication. Acetaminophen 325 mg twice daily for osteoarthritis is not an adequate trial in my opinion before declaring treatment failure. Not only can the NSAID exacerbate CHF, but this gentleman is also on sucralfate which is usually used to treat GI symptoms like GERD or dyspepsia, both of which could be exacerbated by NSAIDs.

Fluid Retention – Additive Effects

On the flip side of the furosemide example above, NSAIDs can have negative synergistic effects with other medications that can worsen edema and fluid retention.

Pregabalin, gabapentin, corticosteroids, pioglitazone, and calcium channel blockers are all common medications that can worsen edema. Patients who take NSAIDs in combination with these medications may be at higher risk of fluid retention. Avoiding these combinations is important and especially important in a patient already requiring diuresis. This is generally a dose-dependent adverse effect so if avoiding these combinations with NSAIDs is not possible, minimizing the dose can be a helpful strategy to reduce the risk of this concern.

Lithium

NSAIDs have the potential to reduce the renal clearance of lithium which can lead to toxicity. Here's a case scenario demonstrating this interaction. A 44 year old male has a past medical history of IBS, bipolar disorder, and depression. Today he presents to an urgent clinic with symptoms of nausea and vomiting. He also states that he feels weak and has been shaky. Upon further investigation, he recently has been complaining of back pain due to an injury at work.

He had a clinic appointment about 2 months ago and his lab work was unremarkable at that time. His lithium level was 0.8. A lithium level was now drawn today and came back at 1.9. Kidney function has remained stable for this patient.

Upon investigating his medication regimen, he has been taking ibuprofen. The lithium NSAID interaction is well known. Lithium is an incredibly important drug for patients who require this medication. There are lots of clinical pearls with this medication and the risk of drug interactions is a very big one. Concentrations of lithium can be elevated by the use of NSAIDs and at a minimum, we need to monitor our patients closely and educate them about the risks of the lithium NSAID interaction.

Antiplatelet Activity

It is well understood that traditional antiplatelet agents like aspirin and clopidogrel are going to increase bleed risk. All NSAIDs have antiplatelet activity which compounds the bleeding risk in those taking both an antiplatelet medication with an NSAID. But what about other drugs that may have less robust platelet inhibition activity like the

SSRIs? The SSRI and NSAID interaction kind of drives me crazy. It is one of those interactions where you don't really know how seriously to take it.

SSRIs have the potential to impact platelet function. NSAIDs have the potential to impact platelet function. The SSRI and NSAID interaction is represented by an increased risk of bleeding with this synergistic effect.

Back to question number one. How seriously do we take this interaction, because it happens all the time? Let me break down my thought process for you and questions you need to consider before making a clinical decision on this interaction.

Are both drugs necessary? In the world of polypharmacy that I live in, getting rid of drugs is a necessity. If we can get rid of one of these drugs, this "problem" is solved. If we can't, we need another idea.

What are the doses and how frequently are patients using them. I'm probably more concerned with a patient on ibuprofen 800 mg TID and sertraline 200 mg than I am with a patient who takes 200 mg of ibuprofen once a month for a headache.

What are their labs? CBC with platelets can help us identify if a patient might be at risk for bleeding and/or demonstrate if they have had blood loss.

Are they displaying any symptoms? Bleeding or bruising is primarily what I am looking for here.

What are their other medications? Are they on an anticoagulant like apixaban or warfarin? If so, I am much more likely to take this seriously and certainly going to try to get them off the NSAID if possible.

Medical history. If this patient has a history of bleeding ulcers, refrain from using an NSAID regardless of the SSRI.

How long have they been on these drugs? If they have done well with the combination without adverse effects, it would be harder to discontinue one of them.

What age is the patient? NSAIDs are less tolerable in the elderly even in the absence of the SSRI.

Which one is the first to go? Usually, depression/anxiety and mental health are more challenging to get under control than pain management, but it is really going to depend upon the patient here.

Is this interaction relevant and how concerned should we be? All in all, I think it is important to recognize that there is potential for a drug interaction here. In the event of a bleed or serious event, in most situations, I'm going to recommend getting off the NSAID to avoid this potential interaction.

In many situations, if the patient's labs are stable and there are no signs/symptoms of blood loss, patients will continue to take these agents together.

NSAIDs and Anticoagulation

NSAIDs are notoriously associated with GI bleeding. Because of their ability to directly damage the GI tract and inhibit the activity of platelets, NSAIDs are the most common medication associated cause of gastrointestinal ulcers. This risk is amplified by the use of warfarin or any other anticoagulant.

The addition of warfarin or any other anticoagulant adds a higher level of bleeding risk when compared to using an NSAID alone. NSAIDs increase the risk of ulceration by a couple of specific mechanisms. COX-1 inhibition accounts for the primary concern of GI bleed risk. All NSAIDs will inhibit COX-1 to varying degrees. In general, the more COX-1 inhibition, the higher the risk for the NSAID to cause GI bleed. Drugs like ketorolac and indomethacin have a higher risk for causing GI bleed.

There are a few strategies that can be used to mitigate the risk of this interaction. The most common method that is selected is to avoid the NSAID and choose alternative analgesic therapy. Because anticoagulation will often be necessary to prevent a high-risk event like a stroke or blood clot, there really isn't much we are likely to do with this medication. Acetaminophen is the most commonly used substitute for mild to moderate pain or acute management of fever. One downside to this strategy is that in the setting of inflammation like rheumatoid arthritis, acetaminophen may not be as effective as NSAIDs.

Assessing the location of pain is important when considering alternatives to oral NSAIDs. Topical formulations remain a viable option for those who have responded well to oral NSAIDs. When the area is limited to small areas like a knee, using a topical NSAID like diclofenac gel is a strong consideration. In general, there is low systemic absorption and risk for GI bleed and other systemic adverse effects is pretty minimal. Cost may be an issue for some patients which is a downside to this option.

On occasion, I have seen other strategies employed. Consideration could be given to a COX-2 inhibitor like celecoxib. Keep in mind that this is not free from risk for GI bleed. In addition, all the other adverse risks of NSAIDs like renal failure and fluid retention still apply with COX-2 inhibitors. Another strategy I have seen used is to place a patient on a PPI for GI protection. This can help reduce the risk of GI bleed. The safest strategy is to avoid NSAIDs altogether when a patient is taking an anticoagulant like apixaban or warfarin.

I also want to caution you about the ease of availability of NSAIDs. Many patients have naproxen or ibuprofen in their medicine cabinets at home and may forget that they shouldn't take these with an anticoagulant. It is so critical to ask about over-the-counter medications and reemphasize education about what the patient should or shouldn't take for pain or fever management.

Opioids

Central Nervous System (CNS) Depressants

CNS depressant interactions are everywhere. Opioids are near the top of the list when it comes to medications that can cause sedation to the point of risking our patient's health. There are so many patients (typically, patients with mental health and pain concerns) on multiple medications that can cause CNS sedation/depression. The list is extensive and includes classes like TCAs, sleepers, opioids, muscle relaxants, benzodiazepines, alcohol, and on and on. There are so many drug combinations that flag this drug interaction on electronic health record programs. Alert fatigue is something that is very real and can put our patients at risk when a clinically significant drug interaction does come our way and in the midst of a busy day, we forget to monitor it appropriately. Here are a few things that I clinically think about when assessing an interaction with two medications that can cause CNS depression.

When I see two CNS depressants used together, the first thing I will look at is the dosing. With the dosing, you need to be able to recognize a high dose versus a low dose. Is oxycodone a total of 10 mg per day or is it 100 mg per day? Is it lorazepam 0.25 mg or 2 mg. The 2 mg dose should scare you a little bit and you should do more follow up especially if it is a new start. In general, the higher the dose, the greater the risk for sedation and overdose.

Benzodiazepines require specific mention when used with opioids. When this combination is used, the risk for respiratory depression and overdose goes up significantly. If this combination is used, I'd strongly encourage a goal to eventually get that patient off this combination. One exception may be in the end-of-life setting. Elderly patients are particularly at risk for complications from medications that can depress the CNS.

Gabapentin and pregabalin use in combination with opioids should also be monitored closely. They are mentioned in the Beers criteria as a potential contributing factor to the risk for opioid overdose and respiratory depression. Minimize dose and avoid the combination if at all possible.

Assessing PRN use is critical. Is the patient using the CNS depressant(s) and how should we advise them to use their PRN medications? If they have an as needed hydrocodone order with alprazolam, it would important to assess their use as well as educate the patient to use extreme caution when using these close together.

What dosing has the patient previously been on? Tolerance is a key concept with the use of opioids. Over time, patients develop tolerance to opioids which may precipitate escalation because the beneficial effects that the patient experienced previously may start to fade. If the patient has tolerated higher doses of medications in the past without issue, they may be less likely to have an issue with a new medication from a similar class. This certainly isn't always true, but it is something to think about.

Additive Effects – Constipation

Opioids are well known for their constipating adverse effects. This can be compounded by the fact that patients may be taking other medications like calcium channel blockers or anticholinergics that can exacerbate this problem. If opioids are necessary in the management of post-op pain, cancer pain, or hospice patients, we will typically manage this adverse effect with laxatives. Ideally, we should work to try to minimize constipation inducing medications over time and as the patient's needs change.

Opioid Antagonism

Opioids can have tremendous withdrawal symptoms that can be awful for patients. In situations of opioid overdose, it is essential that we use opioid antagonists like naloxone. There may be less urgent situations where opioid antagonists may cause some withdrawal symptoms that might go overlooked.

Naltrexone has a unique role in the management of alcohol use disorder. It is an opioid antagonist but has shown benefit in this setting. If opioid abuse or misuse is overlooked in a patient taking naltrexone for alcohol use disorder, it will cause opioid withdrawal. Some symptoms of opioid withdrawal include sweating, anxiety, insomnia, tachycardia, body aches, shakiness, and GI upset.

Hydrocodone

Hydrocodone is most often used in combination with acetaminophen. There are some CYP enzymes that can impact the concentrations of hydrocodone. CYP3A4 and CYP2D6 play a role in the metabolism of hydrocodone. Interestingly, CYP2D6 converts hydrocodone to hydromorphone. This complicates things because hydromorphone has a much more potent opioid effect.

Stronger CYP3A4 inhibitors include medications like clarithromycin, azole antifungals, and some HIV medications. Commonly used medications that have stronger CYP2D6 inhibition include paroxetine, fluoxetine, and bupropion. I think it is important to recognize the potential for alterations in the activity of hydrocodone when a CYP3A4 or CYP2D6 inhibitor is used. It isn't totally understood what the response to a CYP2D6 inhibitor will be, but I think it is an important pathway to remember and recognize that if patients are reporting withdrawal symptoms or symptoms of potential overdose that these interactions could play a significant role.

Oxycodone

Much like hydrocodone, oxycodone could have some impact on drugs that alter the CYP3A4 or CYP2D6 pathway. Be aware if a patient is placed on inducers or inhibitors of these enzymes, that concentrations and clinical activity could increase or decrease. Keep an eye out for signs of toxicity and overdose in patients who have been otherwise stable on their dose of oxycodone.

Tramadol

Tramadol is an opioid medication that can be used for moderate type pain. It is incredibly important to remember that because it has opioid activity, it can certainly lead to the risk of addiction and dependence just like any other opioid. There are some clinical differences with tramadol compared to more traditional opioids like oxycodone or hydrocodone.

One similarity between oxycodone, hydrocodone and tramadol is the metabolic pathway for drug breakdown. CYP3A4 and CYP2D6 are both important pathways. Close attention should be paid to the use of drugs that alter these pathways. Alteration in clinical effectiveness or the risk for toxicity can be impacted by the use of a drug that affects CYP3A4 or CYP2D6.

Seizure and Serotonin Risks

I recall an education session on tramadol and drug abuse and the expert stated that patients addicted to opioids do not like tramadol. One of the primary reasons for this is that tramadol can lower the seizure threshold. As doses of tramadol escalate, which they often do in opioid addiction, the risk for seizures also increases. Be aware of this adverse effect and understand that in patients taking seizure medications or who have a history of seizures, we should do our best to avoid its use.

In addition to the seizure risk of tramadol, tramadol has SNRI activity. This means that it has the potential to be a contributing factor to serotonin syndrome. Here's a case scenario where we look into these risks a little further.

A 74 year old male has been having increasing knee pain. Topical agents have not been effective, acetaminophen doesn't work for him, and NSAIDs are not a good option as he is on warfarin and has kidney disease. His current medication list includes:
- Baby aspirin
- Fluoxetine
- Bupropion
- Omeprazole

- Biotin
- Tramadol
- Phenytoin
- Enalapril
- Nifedipine

In the review of the medication list, it is obviously nice to have doses, but I try to teach the clinical thought process. In this patient, I recognize the fact that he is on phenytoin. Phenytoin is almost exclusively used in the management of seizures. This case highlights one of the tramadol pearls that we just discussed. Tramadol can lower the seizure threshold. This isn't something we worry about too much in patients without a seizure history, but for those who do (or likely have seizures based on the phenytoin), we need to avoid its use or at a minimum be very cautious in using tramadol.

Also of note in this patient is that he is on two medications for depression. I would like to further review this. One of the medications (bupropion) also can contribute to seizure issues. The tramadol and bupropion combination would be a very concerning one to me in a patient who likely has a history of seizures.

I would review the fluoxetine as well. Serotonin syndrome is extremely rare, but tramadol does have the potential to raise serotonergic effects. I would definitely want to know how high of a dose the fluoxetine is as well as assess how much of the tramadol is being used.

Morphine

Inhibition of antiplatelet agents is a concern in a patient with a cardiovascular history requiring a P2Y12 inhibitor. Morphine has been shown to reduce the effectiveness of medications like clopidogrel and prasugrel. While morphine was routinely used for acute coronary syndromes (ACS) in the past, this has changed over the last several years. In ACS it is generally recommended to avoid morphine unless the patient is experiencing substantial pain and one of the major reasons is the fact that it may reduce the effectiveness of antiplatelet therapy.

Codeine

Codeine is well established to be part of the opioid family. The unique aspect of codeine is that its opioid activity is very dependent upon the activity of CYP2D6. Codeine is a classic example of a prodrug and one that I have seen show up on board certification and pharmacology exams numerous times. CYP2D6 is the enzyme that converts codeine to morphine. Morphine is the active metabolite that is primarily responsible for the opioid activity. Any drug that impairs the activity of CYP2D6 will result in less morphine and a reduced clinical response to codeine. Classic common examples of CYP2D6 inhibitors include fluoxetine, paroxetine, and bupropion.

Fentanyl

Fentanyl is a substrate of CYP3A4. This means that numerous clinical interactions can exist. Potent CYP3A4 inhibitors are likely to significantly raise the concentrations of fentanyl which would obviously increase the risk for opioid adverse effects and overdose. CYP3A4 inducers would be likely to do the opposite by reducing concentrations and could potentially contribute to withdrawal symptoms.

Corticosteroids

Blood Sugars – Opposition of Diabetes Medications

Without a doubt, systemic corticosteroids are the most common medications that will oppose the effects of our diabetes medications and raise blood sugars. The most common corticosteroids that I see used in practice are prednisone, prednisolone, triamcinolone, and methylprednisolone. You need to be cautious when starting and discontinuing these agents. Blood sugars will rise with initiation and increases in the dose. Blood sugars can also fall when these agents are discontinued. Here's a case scenario that demonstrates the effect that corticosteroids can have on blood sugar.

About 10 days ago, a 76-year-old male called you to tell you that his spiking blood sugars are higher than they have been in a long time. His blood sugars were in the 300-400 range. He used to never get much above 200. He reports that he has had no diet changes and is adamant that he is taking his insulin as directed.

Because of this change in his blood sugars, his basal insulin was increased from 30 units per day to 35 units per day and 3 days later, increased to 40 units per day as the response from the first increase was inadequate.

Blood sugars did come down back to their usual range, but about 5 days after these changes, he bottomed out and ended up in the emergency room for hypoglycemia.

I think this scenario demonstrates how good history taking can help us identify problems and prevent future problems. He was recently diagnosed with a COPD exacerbation and pneumonia. He was placed on 40 mg of prednisone for 10 days. This prednisone was likely the culprit for the spiking blood sugars.

Once the prednisone was complete, this patient likely could have gone back to his previous insulin dose. If there wasn't a plan to reduce, at a minimum, this patient should have been well educated that blood sugars will likely fall once the prednisone is done.

Immunosuppression

Corticosteroids are well known to be used for specialty purposes as well as for generalized pain and inflammation indications. One of those specialty purposes is for immunosuppression in transplant patients. They are beneficial in preventing organ rejection because corticosteroids can suppress the immune system.

While the immunosuppression is necessary in transplantation, it does mean that patients who are on corticosteroids for any purpose may have an increased risk for infection. This risk may be exacerbated by other medications that can also cause immunosuppression. In oncology, many of the agents that are used will have a negative impact on the immune system and can have an additive effect when used with prednisone. Other immune system modulating agents like azathioprine, methotrexate, and cyclosporine can increase the risk of infection as well. These effects are generally dose and time-dependent. Higher doses and a longer treatment duration may increase the risk of suppressing the immune system.

On the flipside, echinacea is a supplement that may have some immune system stimulating properties. While the clinical literature on preventing upper respiratory tract infections is murky, there is some in vitro data that suggests it may have various immune system stimulating effects. In our patients who are using prednisone for the immunosuppressive purpose of preventive transplant rejection, echinacea should be avoided as there may be potential that it directly opposes immunosuppression.

Vaccines

Because of the immunosuppressive nature of corticosteroids, we have to pay attention when recommending and providing vaccines. The best recommendation is to avoid the concurrent use of corticosteroids and vaccines. If a patient is going to receive an equivalent of 20 mg/day of prednisone or more for longer than 2 weeks, this would be a concern with regards to the use of vaccines. In pediatrics, a prednisone dose of 2mg/kg or higher would be considered immunosuppressive. If a patient has been on this dose and it has been discontinued, the recommended time to wait to begin vaccinations is 3 months following cessation of the corticosteroid. If it is known that a patient is going to be on steroids in the future, it is important to plan vaccination prior to the use of the corticosteroid. It would be important to finish the desired vaccines 2 weeks prior to starting corticosteroids.

CYP3A4 – Prednisone

Prednisone is broken down by CYP3A4. Drugs that inhibit CYP3A4 can increase the concentrations of prednisone. Medications that induce CYP3A4 can lower the concentrations of prednisone. Depending upon what we are trying to do with prednisone, this can be more or less significant. In the setting of immunosuppression to prevent transplant rejection, these interactions are likely more of a concern compared to using it for anti-inflammatory and pain purposes.

Hypokalemia – Diuretics Additive Effect

Prednisone does have a small risk of contributing to hypokalemia. Corticosteroids do this by enhancing renal losses. For me personally, it helps to remember that Addison's disease is due to insufficient levels of endogenous glucocorticoids and mineralocorticoids. One of the risks of this deficiency is hyperkalemia. If we give exogenous or excessive steroids, we could anticipate that the opposite, hypokalemia, could happen. This isn't something that is typically too concerning in patients on low to moderate doses of corticosteroids, but when you have patients who may be predisposed to hypokalemia this risk is going to be a little higher. The most common situation where patients are predisposed to hypokalemia is when they are taking a loop and/or thiazide diuretics.

GI Bleed Risk – NSAIDs

Corticosteroids can be hard on the gut and by themselves may have an increased risk for causing GI bleed. When NSAIDs are added on top of corticosteroids, this risk may be exacerbated even further. I have seen situations where patients have been on both of these medications. In general, it is best to avoid this combination, but if they are used together, we must try to mitigate this risk. Adding a short term PPI for GI protection and avoiding high GI risk NSAIDs like ketorolac and indomethacin would be an important consideration. Celecoxib would likely have less GI risk than tradition NSAIDs.

Edema

Fluid retention and edema can be caused by corticosteroids. It is important to be aware of other agents that may contribute to this adverse effect. NSAIDs, pioglitazone, calcium channel blockers, pregabalin, and gabapentin are all commonly used medications that could enhance this adverse effect of corticosteroids. Limiting doses and duration of therapy of both the prednisone and other agents is a consideration. If the symptoms of swelling, edema, or weight gain are too significant, discontinuation or consideration of alternative agents are also on the table as potential options.

Osteoporosis

Corticosteroids can have additive negative effects on the management of osteoporosis. Be aware of patients who are at risk and medications that may increase the risk of osteoporosis. Excessive thyroid supplementation or using enzyme inducers like phenytoin and carbamazepine may contribute to the risk of osteoporosis. With corticosteroids, the duration of use is more concerning. A patient who receives a 1-2 week course of prednisone is typically not going to be too concerning when it comes to osteoporosis development. The patients we are most concerned about are those that are frequently placed on corticosteroid therapy or those that are taking it chronically.

Cyclobenzaprine

Anticholinergic Burden

Like many other agents we have discussed, cyclobenzaprine is another drug that can have anticholinergic activity. Paying attention to dosing and other agents that have similar activity is critically important to avoid and minimize the risk for anticholinergic adverse effects. These interactions should be especially concerning in our geriatric population.

Primarily because of the anticholinergic nature of cyclobenzaprine, it is listed on the Beers criteria as a potentially harmful medication in the elderly. This drug is even more concerning in patients who are already taking other anticholinergics like oxybutynin, diphenhydramine, hydroxyzine, dicyclomine, or methocarbamol.

So what can we do in place of cyclobenzaprine? Baclofen and tizanidine are two potential options that may be less risky in an elderly patient. In addition, they are typically not considered to have near as much anticholinergic activity as cyclobenzaprine.

Anticholinergic Opposition

In addition to additive anticholinergic effects, it is critical to remember that anticholinergics can reduce the effectiveness of acetylcholinesterase inhibitors like donepezil. Whenever I see these combinations used, I check to see if I can identify when each medication was started. In some cases, the adverse effects of cyclobenzaprine have contributed to a worsening of confusion and dementia. In any situation where we have a patient with dementia, it is critical to check for and avoid the use of anticholinergics whenever possible.

CNS Sedation

In addition to the anticholinergic activity of cyclobenzaprine, it is important to recognize the sedative nature of the medication. Patients with pain concerns often tend to be on numerous other medications that can be sedating. A few common examples of medications that can have additive sedative effects include opioids, gabapentinoids, Z-drugs like zolpidem for sleep, and benzodiazepines.

Serotonergic Interactions

The cyclobenzaprine and SSRI interaction is usually one that flags on drug interaction programs. I'll look at a brief scenario and some questions to ponder.

A 68 year old female was recently prescribed cyclobenzaprine for neck pain. She is also concurrently receiving sertraline 150 mg daily. Cyclobenzaprine has serotonergic properties and if I remember a small bit of chemistry correctly, it is structurally related to the Tri-

Cyclic Antidepressants (TCAs). Because of this, it has some serotonergic activity. Be aware of this and the risk this would pose if the patient is taking other agents that can raise serotonin activity. Here are a few different ways that I might look at handling this interaction.

- The most logical solution in my mind is to change the cyclobenzaprine. It was the medication that was most recently started. With the patient being on sertraline 150 mg I would suspect they have been titrated up on this over months or possibly years. Depending upon what the cyclobenzaprine was prescribed for, that would alter my options. The most common alternatives for muscle relaxant effects would be tizanidine and baclofen. Keep in mind that these agents aren't perfect either as far as adverse effect profiles and drug interaction risk.
- Start low, go slow. If the care team and the patient agree that cyclobenzaprine is appropriate, I'd make sure it was a low dose to start out.
- Another option to consider, depending on how beneficial the sertraline has been, would be to reduce the sertraline dose.
- Use cyclobenzaprine as needed for as short a duration as possible.
- Monitoring/education. When we feel we need to use medications that may be slightly riskier than other options, we need to alert our patients as to what to look for.

Allopurinol

Binding Interactions

The most common interaction you are likely to encounter with allopurinol is the risk of binding interactions. Antacids, in particular, can reduce the absorption of allopurinol. If these medications are given together, this can increase the risk of elevating uric acid. With elevations in uric acid, our patient will be at higher risk for an acute gout flare. The easiest way to avoid this interaction is to not take antacids like calcium carbonate or magnesium hydroxide. That may not always be possible.

In the situation where it is justified to use both an antacid and allopurinol, the easiest way to get around this binding interaction is to alter the timing of administration. Taking allopurinol in the morning and antacids later in the day should not present a problem in altering allopurinol absorption.

144

If a patient has been taking antacids on their own and we want to assess the risk for reduced allopurinol concentrations, there are a couple of ways we can do this. The easiest way is to ask them if they have had any gout flares. If they haven't, then the interaction likely isn't playing too large of a role. Another potential option is to assess a uric acid level and compare it with previous levels. If the uric acid level has gone up, it would be reasonable to assume that the binding interaction could have played some role in elevating that level.

Warfarin

Allopurinol has the potential to raise warfarin concentrations. Because of this, we need to monitor INR more closely following initiation, discontinuation, or dose changes of allopurinol. I think it is also important to note that concentrations of allopurinol may be increased by a reduction in renal function. In a sense, an abrupt change in kidney function could have similar effects to changing the dose. With any drug that interacts with allopurinol, it is important to remember this factor.

Cyclosporine

The allopurinol and cyclosporine interaction is one that isn't as common as other interactions. One of the major reasons is that cyclosporine is a medication that is generally used for a very specialized purpose. Cyclosporine is a calcineurin inhibitor that is primarily used in organ transplantation.

A 58 year old male is receiving chronic cyclosporine for his kidney transplant. He was recently diagnosed with an acute gout flare and elevated uric acid. The long term plan is to manage chronic hyperuricemia with allopurinol. There are a few things to think about here.

Whenever you have a patient on cyclosporine (or tacrolimus), you must review the patient's medication list for drug interactions. There are numerous medications that cyclosporine can impact the concentrations of, or even more challenging, that can alter the levels of cyclosporine.

Allopurinol has been reported to potentially lead to higher levels of cyclosporine. Looking out for potential toxicity and updating the patient's transplant team would be two very important steps in managing this patient.

Also, remember that cyclosporine has the potential to raise uric acid levels. In this type of situation, there probably isn't much we can do to change the cyclosporine because it will likely be 100% necessary, but it is important to remember that fact. We can look at other medications and make sure we aren't using other medications that could raise uric acid levels as well (i.e. thiazide diuretics, niacin, etc.).

Azathioprine and Mercaptopurine

Two other agents that are not commonly used include azathioprine and mercaptopurine. Both are agents that can be used to manage autoimmune diseases like Crohn's and ulcerative colitis. It is important to note that allopurinol can raise the concentrations of both of these drugs. In the case scenario below, I discuss the potential interaction of allopurinol with azathioprine and the risks that may occur because of it.

A 62 year old is taking the following medications
- Enalapril 10 mg daily
- Diclofenac 50 mg twice daily
- Allopurinol 200 mg daily
- Indomethacin 25 mg TID prn
- Azathioprine 50 mg twice daily
- Ranitidine 150 mg at night
- Lansoprazole 15 mg every morning
- Aspirin 81 mg daily
- Metoprolol 25 mg twice daily
- Simvastatin 20 mg daily
- Glipizide 10 mg daily

In this case, allopurinol can potentially increase the concentration of azathioprine, which could potentially lead to toxicity. Symptoms of azathioprine toxicity may manifest as GI symptoms as well as infection if the immune system is suppressed to a large enough extent. The scenario that I have encountered is what to do about this interaction if the patient has been on these medications for a while without issue. The simple answer is to monitor for azathioprine toxicity. The other thing that is important to remember is that changes (dose changes or discontinuation) will potentially change concentrations of the azathioprine.

Drug-Induced Rashes

Allopurinol is one of those medications that is associated with allergic, skin type reactions. There are genetic variations that can significantly raise the risk of this type of reaction. Patients with the genotype HLA-B*58:01 are at higher risk of cutaneous reactions. In addition to genetic variations, there are also drugs that may increase the risk of rash. Be aware that patients who are taking penicillin antibiotics with allopurinol may have a high potential to develop a rash. Patient education and monitoring are important. In addition, if you have had a patient experience rash and they were on this combination, this should be well documented in the medical record.

Bisphosphonates

Binding Interactions

Without a doubt, the most common risk for bisphosphonate interactions is binding interactions. The most commonly used oral bisphosphonates include alendronate, risedronate, and ibandronate. Calcium, iron, magnesium, and other polyvalent cations can bind to these drugs and substantially reduce the absorption. If you recall the pharmacokinetics of oral bisphosphonates, they have extremely low bioavailability and an extremely long half-life.

The easiest way to avoid these interactions is by timing the cations appropriately. Oral bisphosphonates should be administered at least 30-60 minutes prior to all other medications, food or beverage. The only exception for an appropriate beverage is that bisphosphonates should be taken with a full glass of water.

Another method to avoid this interaction is to use alternative pharmacotherapy. Denosumab or IV bisphosphonates are potential options. Remember that it is only oral bisphosphonates that are impacted by the binding interactions.

Esophageal Ulceration

The reason why bisphosphonates should be taken with a full glass of water is to prevent esophageal toxicity. Specifically, the tablet can get stuck in the throat and essentially destroy the tissue in the esophagus. We should be aware of other medications that can increase the risk of esophageal and GI toxicity. NSAIDs are going to be the most commonly used medication that could exacerbate this risk.

Opposition of Beneficial Effects

Be able to recognize medications that may directly oppose the benefit we are trying to provide with bisphosphonates. PPIs, phenytoin, corticosteroids, carbamazepine, and excessive thyroid supplementation may all increase the risk for osteoporosis. Doing what we can to limit the dose and duration of some of these agents is important to try to help reduce the risk for medication-induced osteoporosis.

Tizanidine

CNS Sedation

Like virtually any medication used as a skeletal muscle relaxant, sedation is going to be an adverse effect. It is important to recognize the risk when tizanidine is given with other agents that are sedating. Start low and go slow is one strategy to help avoid over sedating the patient. In addition to this strategy, educating the patient about this risk is important. It would be also advisable to have the patient be cautious about taking sedative medications if they are operating motorized vehicles or machinery. When they first start tizanidine or any other agent that is sedating, encourage the patient to use this medication in the evening or when they know they will be home for a while to ensure that they understand how the medication is going to make them feel.

CYP1A2 Inhibition

Ciprofloxacin and fluvoxamine are two examples of medications that can inhibit CYP1A2. Because CYP1A2 is a critical enzyme for metabolic breakdown of tizanidine, inhibition of this enzyme can result in elevated concentrations of tizanidine leading to the potential for toxicity. Avoidance of this combination would be advisable. In the event the patient doesn't want to change the tizanidine, consider if an alternative to ciprofloxacin might be possible. Assessing pain and switching off of tizanidine is another consideration. If for some odd reason, you cannot change these agents, a dose reduction in the tizanidine would likely be appropriate with close monitoring for signs and symptoms of toxicity.

Clonidine Type Effects

It is important to note that tizanidine is primarily only used for its spasm and pain-relieving purposes, but it is from the alpha-2 agonists class. This is the same class that clonidine is from. Because of this, you need to remember that there may be cardiac and cardiovascular implications with its use.

In patients who are taking beta-blockers or non-dihydropyridine calcium channel blockers, tizanidine has the potential to exacerbate the heart rate lowering effect. Monitoring pulse rate and for symptoms of bradycardia would be important. Have a heightened awareness in those patients who have an existing low or borderline-low heart rate. I would keep a close eye on patients with a baseline heart rate in the 50s to 60s range.

In addition to the potential impact on the pulse, tizanidine can lower blood pressure. Similar to a patient with a borderline low pulse, be aware of patients who have a history of orthostasis or have lower blood pressure. Tizanidine can exacerbate and have additive effects on antihypertensive therapy.

In addition to the above-mentioned effects, recognize that when tizanidine and clonidine are used together, the potential exists for additive effects. In general, I would recommend avoiding this combination if possible. If they must be used together because of limited or unacceptable alternatives, close monitoring, and cautious initiation and titration would be appropriate.

Baclofen

CNS Depressant

The drug interaction potential with baclofen is generally a little less than compared to tizanidine. The overwhelming percentage of drug interactions involving baclofen will be of the CNS depressant type. As we have discussed with numerous other CNS depressant medications, reducing doses, avoiding concomitant use, and patient monitoring are incredibly important considerations.

Additive Effects

Two adverse effects that may show up on account of baclofen use include constipation and hypotension. Be aware of patients who are taking agents that could have additive effects.

Hydroxychloroquine

Immunosuppression

Hydroxychloroquine has the potential to raise the concentrations of cyclosporine. Because cyclosporine and other specialty transplant immunosuppressive agents aren't commonly used in family practice, if you ever see an order for one or know you are working with a transplant patient, I would strongly recommend that you look up potential drug interactions each time a new medication is going to be initiated.

In addition, if there are questions pertaining to the effect that it will have on any medication being used for transplant purposes, it would be advisable to involve the specialists that are working with that patient on their transplant management.

Hypoglycemia Risk

Hydroxychloroquine has been associated with hypoglycemia. We need to pay close attention to this in our patients with diabetes. I would focus most of your attention on those patients who are using insulin or sulfonylureas. In addition, recognizing the patient's past medical history is important. If they have a history of hypoglycemia episodes, this would raise additional flags and necessitate even closer monitoring if hydroxychloroquine is necessary.

QTc Prolongation

While hydroxychloroquine is not likely to cause QTc prolongation on its own, be aware of its potential to add to the cumulative risk. Patients taking amiodarone or other antiarrhythmics would be at the highest risk.

Retinal Toxicity

Hydroxychloroquine is a unique medication in that one of the adverse effects is retinopathy. This risk for retinopathy can be exacerbated by tamoxifen. Because of this risk, it is recommended that patients taking chronic hydroxychloroquine have routine eye assessments with an ophthalmologist.

Hepatotoxicity

Methotrexate is a medication used in oncology, but I'm going to focus my education more so on areas where methotrexate is used in the management of auto-immune diseases like rheumatoid arthritis and psoriasis. Methotrexate is sometimes used in combination with other agents that may cause hepatotoxicity. Drugs like leflunomide, hydroxychloroquine, and sulfasalazine carry a small risk of hepatotoxicity, but can potentially have additive type risks when used in combination with methotrexate.

In addition, recall that patients with a history of alcoholism will also be at risk for hepatotoxicity. In addition, patients taking acetaminophen, amiodarone, and isoniazid can have an increased risk of liver dysfunction. Close monitoring of LFTs can help identify abnormalities and increases from baseline in the event that hepatotoxic agents need to be used together.

NSAIDS

NSAIDs have the potential to raise the concentrations of methotrexate. There is a scenario where these medications are used together in clinical practice. The most common situation where these medications will be used together is in the setting of a rheumatoid arthritis flare. Recognize and potentially monitor for some of the risks associated with methotrexate toxicity such as hepatotoxicity, nausea, vomiting, mucositis, neutropenia, immunosuppression, and thrombocytopenia in patients who need to add an NSAID for acute pain relief.

Antibiotics

Much like the NSAIDs, Bactrim (trimethoprim/sulfamethoxazole) has the potential to raise concentrations of methotrexate. As mentioned before, assessing for the risk of hematologic toxicity and hepatotoxicity should be considered. There are exceptions, but with both NSAIDs and even more so sulfamethoxazole/trimethoprim, we are likely to only use these medications for short term purposes. If that is the case, the interaction timeframe will be limited.

In addition to trimethoprim/sulfamethoxazole, some of the cephalosporins, penicillins, tetracyclines, and quinolone antibiotics may increase the risk of methotrexate toxicity.

151

Vaccines

Similar to corticosteroids, methotrexate can potentially blunt the immune response. This is very important to recognize in the setting of vaccination. Let's think about an example.

A 44 year old is newly diagnosed with rheumatoid arthritis and it is determined that methotrexate therapy is going to be indicated and initiated. In this situation, you would want to review vaccination status and ideally give those vaccines 2 weeks prior to starting the methotrexate to ensure a robust immune response and maximize potential benefit from the vaccines. It is important to note that it will not harm the patient to give them an inactivated vaccine while they are taking methotrexate or any other immunosuppressive agent, but the effectiveness is likely to decline as immunosuppression increases.

Overall, the class of penicillin antibiotics has a pretty low risk for drug interactions. And even when there are drug interactions, the intensity and severity of those interactions are likely to be low. There aren't many situations where you would outright avoid the use of amoxicillin or another penicillin antibiotic because of drug interactions.

Warfarin

There are numerous antibiotics that can cause problems for warfarin. It is difficult to predict what is going to happen to an INR when an antibiotic is started and this is due to various factors. Type of infection, dietary changes, direct drug effects on concentrations, and alteration in the normal gut flora can all potentially impact the activity of warfarin. In nearly all cases with antibiotics, the most likely occurrence is for the INR to go up. This possibility is a reality with penicillin antibiotics. Checking an INR after initiation and discontinuation is an appropriate measure to manage this drug interaction.

Vaccines

There are some unique vaccines that can have their effectiveness reduced due to the use of certain antibiotics. Typhoid vaccine and cholera vaccine effectiveness can both be compromised due to amoxicillin or other antibiotics. This interaction is true of the majority of antibiotics and I won't touch on it much further than in the penicillin section. This is usually easily avoided as most of the time antibiotics are used only for short term purposes. So ensuring that the drug is out of systemic circulation when the vaccination is given is pretty easy to accomplish. I think the most important pearl to recognize is that if someone is considering using the typhoid or cholera vaccine, be aware that many antibiotics can impact the effectiveness.

Allopurinol and Methotrexate Toxicity

The risk of rash and allergic reaction are a possibility with penicillin antibiotics. I discussed in the allopurinol section how this combination can increase the risk of drug-induced rash. With the use of methotrexate, it was also discussed how many antibiotics can raise concentrations of the drug. Penicillin antibiotics like amoxicillin are no exception.

Birth Control

I recall learning years ago that amoxicillin and other penicillin antibiotics can reduce the therapeutic effectiveness of birth control, essentially leaving a patient at risk for pregnancy. This was based upon anecdotal case reports.

We do now have evidence that this interaction does not increase the risk of pregnancy. I still have heard of providers and other pharmacists educate about this potential interaction despite stronger evidence indicating that it should not be an issue. No matter what your comfort level with the evidence is, it would likely not harm your patients to tell them to abstain from sexual activity during the course of a penicillin antibiotic. When educating patients, a prudent approach is to educate them that there have been case reports of this happening, but the overwhelming majority of sound clinical evidence is that this interaction is not significant.

Macrolide Antibiotics

QTc Prolongation

Azithromycin, clarithromycin, and erythromycin are the most commonly used macrolide antibiotics. Of the three, azithromycin is much more commonly used. QTc prolongation is a potential risk with all three of these agents. This is a challenging interaction to handle. Patients will typically take azithromycin for less than a week. Because of this very short duration, it is difficult to monitor and challenging to know how much monitoring should be done. With any medication and the risk for QT prolongation, it is important to look at the risk factors that may be associated with a patient and determine how aggressive we need to be in monitoring. One of the more important factors is whether they are on any other QT-prolonging drugs like amiodarone. Another point of emphasis should be on reviewing a baseline EKG to determine whether or not further monitoring or an alteration of the drug regimen needs to be done.

P-glycoprotein Inhibitors

Macrolides have the potential for drug interactions by inhibiting P-glycoprotein. Dabigatran is an anticoagulant that can have its active metabolite be affected by P-glycoprotein inhibition. For example, if a macrolide antibiotic is used with dabigatran, it can significantly increase concentrations and increase the blood-thinning effect of the active metabolite. Because of this risk, dose reductions might be considered while the patient is on the antibiotic. Alternative antibiotics might be considered if there is one that would be less likely to interact and effectively treats the infection we are trying to manage. Many will simply elect to have the patient monitor for signs and symptoms of bruising or bleeding. Just like with QTc prolongation, the short duration of therapy for antibiotics makes this and many other interactions challenging to navigate.

There is some minor evidence that drugs like the macrolides could slightly raise the concentrations of more commonly used anticoagulants like apixaban and rivaroxaban. No dosage changes are recommended due to this interaction, but it makes sense to recognize the minor risk particularly if the patient is reporting an increase in bruising or bleeding.

Clarithromycin

Clarithromycin isn't used very often. When it is used, it is most often used in the treatment of Helicobacter Pylori. One of the major reasons it isn't used very often is due to drug interactions. Clarithromycin is well known for being a potent CYP3A4 inhibitor. Because of this, it is contraindicated with many common medications. Both lovastatin and simvastatin are contraindicated with clarithromycin. This combination would lead to a substantial elevation in the concentration of the statin and increase the risk for rhabdomyolysis.

In addition to the action of CYP3A4 inhibition, clarithromycin can affect P-glycoprotein as mentioned above. Because of the 3A4 and P-glycoprotein activity, we have to be aware that this can raise the concentrations of two commonly used anticoagulants like apixaban and rivaroxaban.

Other commonly used medications that may be affected by CYP3A4 and/or P-glycoprotein inhibition include calcium channel blockers, aripiprazole, carbamazepine, atorvastatin, alprazolam, amiodarone, quetiapine, trazodone, and many more.

I think the most important educational point to remember with clarithromycin, is if you ever use it, you have to recognize that there will likely be drug interactions. Be sure to assess for this prior to using the medication.

Erythromycin

The major reason why azithromycin is typically used more frequently than other macrolide antibiotics is because it has less significant drug interaction than clarithromycin and erythromycin. In general, erythromycin is seldom used as an antibiotic because it is going to have many of the same overlapped inhibitory effects on CYP3A4 as clarithromycin. It is pretty seldom that you will see erythromycin used because of the drug interaction risks.

Rarely, you may see it used for its prokinetic ability. Patients with gastroparesis may get some relief with the use of erythromycin, but you have to be extremely careful to assess for the risk of drug interactions. If using erythromycin for prokinetic purposes, it is important to assess a patient's medication list to ensure that we aren't using medications like anticholinergics that can oppose the motility of the gut and the benefit you are trying to provide by using erythromycin.

Metronidazole

Metronidazole has a few relevant clinical uses. It can be used in the setting of various intra-abdominal infections, Helicobacter pylori, bacterial vaginosis, and possibly as an alternative for a Clostridium difficile infection.

Alcohol

Alcohol is rarely a good idea in combination with any medication. Metronidazole in combination with alcohol is a special kind of absolute no-no. It is well known to be associated with a disulfiram reaction. Symptoms from this reaction include flushing, tachycardia, nausea and vomiting, and dizziness. You must educate your patients about this risk. Alcohol should absolutely be avoided in combination with metronidazole.

In a patient who is using injectable or rectal forms of medications, it is very important to remember the entire components of products, not just the active ingredients. Medications containing propylene glycol can cause a disulfiram reaction when your patient is also receiving metronidazole. Some commonly used injectable or rectal products that may contain propylene glycol include lorazepam, diazepam, phenytoin, and sulfamethoxazole.

Warfarin

Metronidazole has some inhibitory action on CYP2C9 which is an important enzyme in breaking down S-warfarin. When metronidazole is used, it can prevent the breakdown of warfarin and ultimately increase concentrations. This will increase bleeding risk. Checking INR, monitoring our patient for the risk of bleeding or bruising, and avoiding metronidazole are all potential options in managing this interaction. I shared a case example in the warfarin section regarding this interaction.

Quinolone Antibiotics

Quinolone use has come under more scrutiny over the years due to their adverse effect profile. However, their drug interaction risk should not be overlooked. Two of the most common drug interactions include QTc prolongation risk and binding interactions.

Levofloxacin – QTc Prolongation

You have to be aware that when levofloxacin is used with amiodarone, there is a significant risk for QTc prolongation. In general, using this combination together should be avoided. Looking at alternatives for the levofloxacin is going to be your most likely path to avoid this interaction. There have been numerous case reports of this interaction leading to Torsades de Pointes. Interestingly, ciprofloxacin doesn't seem to have as much risk in QTc prolongation. Although we would still want to assess for risk factors of QTc prolongation like preexisting heart disease, hypokalemia, baseline EKG, hypomagnesemia, using ciprofloxacin with amiodarone may be a possibility.

Binding Interactions

Treatment failure with quinolone antibiotics is a real possibility when we don't pay attention to these interactions. Calcium, magnesium, iron, and sucralfate are a few of the more common medications and supplements that will reduce the concentrations of quinolone antibiotics. If holding the supplements doesn't present an immediate concern for the patient's health, this is usually the easiest path to take. If the medication that is causing the binding interaction is deemed necessary, adjusting the timing of those medications is critical. In general, taking the quinolone antibiotic 2 hours before or 4-6 hours after the interacting medication will help substantially to reduce the potential for any reduction in absorption.

Because many patients will take supplements without approval of their provider or pharmacist, you have to specifically ask about the use of supplements. In some cases, quinolone absorption can be reduced by as much as 50-75% when used with a drug that will bind to it. Here's a case scenario where these binding interactions may have contributed to "recurrent pneumonia" and excessive use of antibiotics.

GF is a 77 year old male with a past medical history of BPH, COPD, hypertension, constipation, Barrett's esophagus, and anemia. Of late, he has had recurrent pneumonia episodes requiring frequent antibiotic use. He has had 3 courses of antibiotics within the last four months to treat pneumonia.

His current medication list includes:
- Aspirin 81 mg daily
- Proscar 5 mg daily
- Doxazosin 2 mg daily
- Tiotropium once daily
- Advair 500/50 BID
- Metoprolol 50 mg BID
- Hydrochlorothiazide 25 mg daily
- Lisinopril 2.5 mg daily
- Senna S 1 tab BID
- Ferrous sulfate 325 mg BID
- Omeprazole 40 mg BID

Recent antibiotics used and now completed were; amoxicillin/azithromycin combination, doxycycline, and levofloxacin. Respiratory symptoms seem to have resolved, but he is currently complaining of watery diarrhea.

With increasing diarrhea and recent, persistent antibiotic use, it is hard to ignore the possibility of C. diff. Testing should likely be considered. The other factor that we may or may not be able to do anything about is the use of the PPI. PPIs can increase the risk of C. diff, but there is also a concern with Barrett's esophagus. A careful risk/benefit would have to be looked at.

With the recurrent respiratory infection and use of doxycycline and levofloxacin, I would look into the past history and try to find out if the patient was taking (or holding) iron appropriately with these two medications. Binding interactions are much more common when patients are taking interacting medications multiple times per day and not paying attention to the timing of administration.

Ciprofloxacin

In addition to the previously mentioned interactions, ciprofloxacin can inhibit CYP1A2. There are a few medications where this is a concern. Antipsychotics like clozapine and olanzapine can have their concentrations raised by CYP1A2 inhibitors. In addition, the skeletal muscle relaxant, tizanidine, can also have an exponential increase in concentrations. Theophylline is an older medication that is notorious for drug interactions. Zolpidem for sleep is another commonly used medication that can have concentrations raised by ciprofloxacin. By inhibiting CYP1A2, ciprofloxacin can increase the risk of theophylline toxicity. While this interaction is very clinically significant, the likelihood of encountering a patient on theophylline is extremely low due to its narrow therapeutic index window and negative adverse effect profile. Like theophylline, caffeine is also broken down by CYP1A2. In patients who are prescribed ciprofloxacin, be aware of the risk for tachycardia, insomnia, and anxiety associated with elevated caffeine concentrations.

Sulfamethoxazole/Trimethoprim

Sulfa Allergy

One of the easiest and most important assessments prior to starting a medication is to review the patient's allergy list. This is something that I have seen overlooked numerous times in my career. I've personally made this mistake which I discuss in my book *Pharmacotherapy: Clinical Pharmacy Pearls, Case Studies, and Common Sense.* The sulfa allergy can be a challenging one if documentation is inaccurate, inadequate, and the patient doesn't remember what happened. Sulfamethoxazole is the quintessential example of a "sulfa" drug and when the patient reports a "sulfa" allergy, this is typically what they are referring to. I can't emphasize enough the importance of careful history taking and documentation when assessing the risk for drug/allergy interactions.

Phenytoin and Warfarin

Phenytoin and warfarin are two high-risk medications that can be impacted by the use of sulfamethoxazole/trimethoprim. Both of these interactions are likely due in part by activity on CYP2C9.

Here's a case scenario involving phenytoin and sulfamethoxazole/trimethoprim:

An 81-year-old female has a history of GERD, OA, and seizures. She hasn't been feeling the best and reports fatigue and painful urination. She has experienced this before and believes she has a urinary tract infection. A urinalysis is ordered and her final diagnosis is a UTI.

Her medications include phenytoin 200 mg twice daily, ranitidine 150 mg daily, and acetaminophen 500 mg three times daily.

For her UTI, she is prescribed Bactrim (sulfamethoxazole/trimethoprim) twice daily for 10 days.

Prior to the Bactrim Rx, she has been seizure-free for seven years. Her most recent phenytoin level was from 6 months ago and was 15.9. Prior to the symptoms stemming from the UTI, she was doing well and displaying no signs of phenytoin toxicity.

On day 5 of the 10-day course of sulfamethoxazole/trimethoprim, she begins feeling dizzy, lethargic and her husband reports that she is more confused. In addition, the husband mentioned that she has been slurring her speech more. The husband feels that she is having a stroke and takes her to the emergency department. Upon assessment, a phenytoin level was checked and came back at 26.8.

With the sulfamethoxazole/trimethoprim and phenytoin interaction, inhibition of CYP enzymes is likely at play. Trimethoprim can inhibit CYP2C8 and CYP2C9 which play a role in phenytoin metabolism. Because of this inhibition, the concentration of phenytoin can rise and result in toxicity.

Methotrexate

Under the methotrexate section, we did discuss the potential for methotrexate concentrations to be increased by sulfamethoxazole/trimethoprim. In addition to the potential to enhance the risk of methotrexate toxicity, also remember that trimethoprim is known to contribute to folic acid deficiency. Because of this fact, the use of trimethoprim may directly oppose the benefit we are trying to provide by giving folic acid supplementation with methotrexate. This is likely not a concern in patients who are taking a traditional course of sulfamethoxazole/trimethoprim for acute infection and more likely a concern in patients who may be taking long term antibiotic prophylaxis.

Hyperkalemia

Recall that trimethoprim may have some activity similar to potassium-sparing diuretics. Because of this, we have to be aware of the potential for hyperkalemia. This was discussed previously with a case study that demonstrated this risk. It is important to monitor potassium levels in patients who may be on other potassium elevating agents like ACE inhibitors, potassium-sparing diuretics and ARBs or at risk for hyperkalemia such as in CKD.

Cephalosporins

Cephalosporins are a very broad category of medications. In general, they are pretty well tolerated and many will have a similar drug interaction profile to the penicillin antibiotics. I'm going to focus on two that are very commonly used in practice: cephalexin and ceftriaxone.

Zinc

Cephalexin is an oral antibiotic, and binding interactions are possible. The most common supplement that can reduce the concentrations of cephalexin is zinc. Holding the zinc while cephalexin is being used is the simplest way to manage this interaction. Altering the timing of administration is another way. Iron and calcium do not seem to be as problematic with the use of cephalexin. Ceftriaxone obviously doesn't have this concern as we avoid the oral route.

Vaccines

Much like the penicillin antibiotics, cephalosporins can have a negative impact on the efficacy of certain vaccines. Typhoid vaccine and cholera vaccine effectiveness can both be compromised due to cephalosporins. This is usually easily avoided as most of the time antibiotics are used only for short term purposes. So ensuring that the drug is out of systemic circulation when the vaccination is given is pretty easy to accomplish.

Warfarin

The same impact that penicillin antibiotics can have on the risk of raising INRs in patients taking warfarin can happen with cephalosporins. As with many other antibiotics, it is difficult to predict what is going to happen to an INR when an antibiotic like cephalexin is started. Type of infection, dietary changes, direct drug effects on concentrations, and alteration in the normal gut flora can all potentially impact the activity of warfarin. In nearly all cases with antibiotics, the most likely occurrence is for the INR to go up. Checking an INR after initiation and discontinuation of a cephalosporin is an appropriate measure to manage this drug interaction.

Tetracyclines

Doxycycline is by far the most commonly used tetracycline antibiotic. Tetracycline, demeclocycline, and minocycline use in clinical practice is much less common. Because of this, I'm going to primarily focus on doxycycline, but many interactions will impact the entire class of tetracycline antibiotics.

Binding Interactions

Treatment failure with tetracycline antibiotics is a real possibility when we don't pay attention to these interactions. Calcium, magnesium, iron, and sucralfate are a few of the more common medications and supplements that will reduce the concentrations of tetracycline antibiotics. If holding the supplements doesn't present an immediate concern for the patient's health, this is usually the easiest path to take. If the medication that is causing the binding interaction is deemed necessary, adjusting the timing of those medications is critical. In general, taking the tetracycline antibiotic 2 hours before or 4-6 hours after the interacting medication will help substantially reduce the potential for any reduction in absorption.

Phenytoin

On account of its enzyme induction, phenytoin is likely to lead to lower concentrations of doxycycline. Because of this, we have to be aware that treatment failure is a possibility. I would look to alternative agents to treat an infection in an attempt to avoid the risk of lower doxycycline concentrations. Changing phenytoin is likely not going to be an option. Altering the timing of administration will likely not have an impact as doxycycline is dosed twice per day, and the duration of activity of phenytoin is going to be going on all throughout the day. If it didn't phenytoin likely wouldn't be effective at managing seizures.

Warfarin

Like many of the other antibiotics discussed, tetracycline derivatives can potentially raise INR. The level of significance is not the same as sulfamethoxazole/trimethoprim or metronidazole, but it is likely going to warrant closer monitoring of the INR.

Additive Effects – Sun Sensitivity

Tetracycline antibiotics are notorious for increasing the risk of sun sensitivity. Patients need to be extremely careful about sun exposure and the risk of sunburn while taking these medications. This can be exacerbated in a patient who is taking other medications that may cause similar effects. Diuretics, retinoids, and sulfonamides are a few common examples of medications that could increase the risk of sun sensitivity. Quinolone antibiotics and trimethoprim can contribute as well, but it would be unlikely that the patient would be taking two different antibiotics at the same time.

Clindamycin

An easy error for a rookie is to mistake clindamycin for clarithromycin. Clindamycin is not a macrolide antibiotic and has a different spectrum of coverage. Clindamycin is also different from the macrolides in that it has a much lower risk for drug interactions in general.

CYP3A4 Inducers

One of the major interactions of clindamycin is an interaction that can occur with many other drugs. The extent of the interaction is not huge, but CYP3A4 inducers have the potential to lower concentrations of clindamycin. Because of this, antibiotic failure is a possibility. We probably aren't going to do much about this interaction other than to be aware of it. Classic CYP3A4 inducers include phenytoin, rifampin, carbamazepine, primidone, and phenobarbital.

Enzyme Induction – CYP3A4

I would consider CYP3A4 the most consequential enzyme that rifampin induces. The clinical impact of using a drug like rifampin is real. Fortunately, the frequency of use in clinical practice is relatively low. I've only seen it used a handful of times in 10+ years of practice. When I see it being used, it is definitely one of those medications that I look up every medication the patient is taking and run a drug interaction screen.

Common CYP3A4 interactions include effects on medications like diltiazem, verapamil, apixaban, rivaroxaban, atorvastatin, amiodarone, simvastatin, and warfarin. In the overwhelming majority of situations, adding rifampin to a patient's regimen will likely cause subtherapeutic concentrations.

It can reduce the concentrations of many medications, increasing the risk for treatment failure. In addition to this concern, whenever a change in dose is made, concentrations can fluctuate.

Discontinuation can be as concerning as starting the medication. Here's a case scenario that demonstrates that risk.

The patient was placed on rifampin for osteomyelitis. An important fact about osteomyelitis is that it is an infection that generally takes a long time to treat. What ended up happening was that the Coumadin (warfarin) the individual was on needed to be escalated to above 15 mg per day because rifampin is an enzyme inducer (remember it causes many drugs to be chewed up faster). Following the escalation of the dose to overcome the enzyme induction, the patient's INR was stabilized.

When the rifampin was stopped, it was inevitable that a surplus of warfarin was going to happen without a reduction in dose and close monitoring of the INR. The rifampin was discontinued shortly after previous INR was about 2.1 and 30 days after that good INR (treating Afib), the INR came back at 9.6.

This is a great reminder that drug interactions can have a clinical impact not only when new drugs are started or increased but also when drugs are discontinued.

P-glycoprotein Induction

Rifampin's ability to induce P-glycoprotein plays a critical role in altering many of the direct oral anticoagulants. Apixaban and rivaroxaban concentrations can be reduced on account of p-glycoprotein induction. P-glycoprotein induction in combination with CYP3A4 induction makes the use of apixaban or rivaroxaban contraindicated with the use of rifampin.

CYP2C19 Induction

Clopidogrel can be impacted by the use of rifampin. Rifampin can induce CYP2C19. CYP2C19 is the enzyme necessary to activate clopidogrel. When starting enzyme inducers like rifampin, we are likely going to cause lower concentrations and reduced effectiveness of the other medication. This is a situation where the opposite can happen. With CYP2C19 induction, it can create more of the active metabolite of clopidogrel. This can lead to an increased risk of bleeding in our patients taking this combination.

CYP2C9 Induction

In addition to effects on CYP3A4, 2C19, and P-glycoprotein, rifampin has enzyme-inducing effects on CYP2C9. This can have significant impacts on a drug like Bactrim. Warfarin metabolism is also dependent upon CYP2C9. Lower concentrations of both of these agents would be likely in a patient taking rifampin. Here's a case scenario where induction of CYP2C9 and possibly CYP2C19 have impacted the concentration of phenytoin.

A 47 year old patient with diabetes and seizure disorder is diagnosed with new-onset osteomyelitis. The patient's seizures were well controlled on phenytoin as they had not had one in well over a year. The latest total phenytoin level was 11.

As part of the antibiotic regimen for the osteomyelitis, the patient is placed on rifampin. Within 3 weeks of starting rifampin, the patient had a seizure. At the time of the seizure, the labs were checked and revealed a substantial deviation from previous phenytoin levels. The phenytoin level was 6.7 likely due to the rifampin and phenytoin interaction as the patient had been previously well controlled.

It was decided that the dose of phenytoin would be increased with close monitoring for toxicity as well as for seizures. They wanted to stay on top of the levels, so it was elected to check the phenytoin level on a weekly basis. This allowed for adequate monitoring when the course of rifampin for osteomyelitis had been completed.

Liver Toxicity

Rifampin has been associated with liver toxicity. Because of this, be aware of other agents that may have cumulative effects on the liver. Isoniazid is a medication that is often used in tuberculosis care. It is associated with liver toxicity and may increase the risk when used in combination with rifampin. Patient monitoring of liver function combined with assessing for signs and symptoms of liver toxicity would be appropriate in an interaction like this. We'd also like to ensure that other liver toxic agents are not used. Specifically, patient use of alcohol should be avoided and strongly discouraged.

Nitrofurantoin

Nitrofurantoin is almost exclusively used in the treatment and possibly prophylaxis of UTI's. It doesn't use traditional liver mechanisms for breakdown, so drug interactions via the CYP enzyme systems aren't a concern. There only a few minor concerns to be aware of.

Hyperkalemia

Hyperkalemia has been reported in patients who are taking an aldosterone antagonist like spironolactone. The risk is pretty low, and I cannot recall the last time I have seen a provider check a potassium level in a patient who was prescribed this combination. I'd review a few things before considering whether or not to check a potassium level after starting nitrofurantoin in a patient taking spironolactone.

I'd first look at the patient's baseline potassium level. If it is moderate to lower end of normal (i.e. 3.5-4.0 mEq/L) and the patient has no other risk factors for hyperkalemia, most would probably not consider checking a level as the risk of hyperkalemia would likely be extremely low. Some other factors that I might consider is if that patient has a history of hyperkalemia, is taking other potassium elevating medications, or has chronic kidney disease.

Valacyclovir and Acyclovir

Vaccines

One of the best ways to combat viral infections is through vaccines. Valacyclovir and acyclovir can be helpful in managing certain acute infections such as varicella, but they can also stifle the activity of the varicella vaccine (Varivax). Because Varivax is a live vaccine these antiviral agents will reduce the immune response to the vaccine and leave patients more susceptible to future infections. The easiest way to avoid the risk of this interaction is to not use valacyclovir or acyclovir near the time of the vaccination.

CYP1A2

Valacyclovir and acyclovir can have some modest impact on CYP1A2. If you recall from earlier in this chapter, we discussed ciprofloxacin. Much like ciprofloxacin, these antiviral agents can increase concentrations of certain medications by the inhibition of CYP1A2. Tizanidine, clozapine, and theophylline are examples of drugs that could head toward toxic levels if given with these antivirals. If adverse reactions are encountered on account of this drug interaction, we are likely going to look at reducing the doses of those agents.

It is important to recognize that acyclovir comes in the form of a topical agent as well as the traditional oral formulation. Systemic absorption is likely not going to be significant enough to cause interactions with vaccination and CYP1A2.

Fluconazole

If you are ever considering using fluconazole or see an order for its use, you must recognize that there are numerous drug interactions. Primary concerns for drug interactions include its effects on numerous CYP enzymes as well as the potential for QTc prolongation. Let's break them down.

CYP3A4

By now, I hope I've demonstrated that there are a lot of drugs that are broken down by CYP3A4 If you haven't got the message yet, I'll remind you. Here's a list of common drugs that can be significantly affected by alterations in the CYP3A4 system. Amiodarone, colchicine, fentanyl, atorvastatin, simvastatin, lovastatin, carbamazepine, alprazolam, aripiprazole, diltiazem, warfarin, verapamil, tacrolimus, and cyclosporine.

Since fluconazole inhibits the activity of CYP3A4, concentrations of any of these medications can be increased leading to the potential for adverse effects.

CYP2C9

While there is a lower total number of drugs that are impacted by the CYP2C9 enzyme, there are some heavy hitters that can result in substantial harm for our patients. Warfarin is substantially broken down by CYP2C9. This inhibition in combination with CYP3A4 inhibition can strongly reduce the metabolism of warfarin and lead to big elevations in INR. In addition to warfarin, many sulfonylureas and phenytoin can be impacted by CYP2C9 inhibition. Both agents can obviously have devastating adverse effects if concentrations become too high. Here's a case scenario of the fluconazole phenytoin interaction.

A 64 year old female with a history of seizures, hypertension, and osteoarthritis was diagnosed with a case of recurrent vaginal candidiasis. Her current medications included:
- Phenytoin
- Enalapril
- Amlodipine
- Ibuprofen as needed

Her previous labs were unremarkable with a total Dilantin (phenytoin) level of 16 and seizure-free for well over a period of a year. She had not been experiencing any signs of toxicity as well.

For the treatment of the candidiasis, she was prescribed Diflucan (fluconazole) for a period of 14 days. Approximately halfway through the treatment period, the family was concerned with a change in mentation in the patient. She also had a fall and was having trouble walking. The family was questioning if the patient was having side effects from the newly prescribed fluconazole.

Upon investigation, a phenytoin level was checked and revealed to be 27. She was diagnosed with phenytoin toxicity.

When I think of fluconazole, I normally think of all the classic CYP3A4 interactions. The phenytoin and fluconazole interaction is likely caused by fluconazole's ability to inhibit CYP2C9.

CYP2C19

Because of fluconazole's ability to inhibit CYP2C19, there's a couple of different interactions I've run into in clinical practice. The first one is cilostazol. Cilostazol is broken down by CYP2C19. With the use of fluconazole, cilostazol's concentrations are going to be increased.

168

Another clinically relevant interaction with clopidogrel was mentioned before, but I will discuss it in more detail here. Let's review a case scenario and talk about some strategies to manage the interaction between fluconazole and clopidogrel.

A 59 year old male with oropharyngeal candidiasis is prescribed fluconazole 100 mg daily for 14 days. He is currently taking clopidogrel. Clopidogrel is a prodrug that is metabolized to its active form by CYP2C19. Fluconazole can inhibit this enzyme potentially leading to lower concentrations of the active metabolite and ultimately reduced effectiveness. Whether this matters and how much it matters clinically is the million-dollar question that no one will likely be able to perfectly predict. However, there are some critical questions that we can ask to potentially avoid this combination or minimize the risk of problems due to the interaction.

The first question I would like to assess: Is there an alternative to fluconazole? There may not be, but in this situation assessing if something like topical clotrimazole or nystatin is an option would likely be my first step. If fluconazole is absolutely necessary, I would inquire about the severity of the infection and the possibility of limiting the duration to 7 days and reassess.

Is clopidogrel warranted long term? Depending upon the indication, clopidogrel may not be being used for the long term. Was the patient only supposed to be on clopidogrel for 12 months? If we are close to that timeframe this strategy might be considered. In this unlikely, yet convenient event where the patient is approaching the end of therapy and fluconazole is necessary, clopidogrel could potentially be discontinued.

Consider an alternative to clopidogrel? This isn't really high on my list to change a likely long term drug due to a short term drug, but the thought crossed my mind to consider prasugrel. Also, looking at if the patient is on aspirin and the indication for clopidogrel would be significantly important if looking at changing up clopidogrel.

The last option is to do nothing. When it comes to drug interactions, this is often a choice that is made. It is pretty hard to monitor for a drug interaction like this one because if we are wrong and we should have done something, there is a very small chance that a really bad thing could happen (i.e. heart attack or stroke).

QTc Prolongation

In addition to its effects on many CYP enzymes, fluconazole has been associated with QTc prolongation. In many cases, the CYP interactions and intrinsic QTc prolongation of fluconazole can work together to raise the QTc interval substantially.

Let's take amiodarone for example. Many drugs can have additive effects on QTc prolongation. Levofloxacin, ondansetron, and citalopram are a few common examples. Fluconazole can have this effect as well but with the added potential of significant CYP3A4 inhibition, it can raise the concentrations of amiodarone, thus further enhancing the possibility for QT prolongation. Although maybe to a slightly less significant extent, the same thing can happen when using fluconazole with an antipsychotic like aripiprazole.

Gabapentinoids, gabapentin and pregabalin, are commonly used agents in the setting of various types of nerve pain. Fortunately, they are fairly low risk when it comes to the risk of drug interactions. They have virtually no impact on the CYP enzymes which is excellent for avoiding interactions. Their primary interactions involve additive adverse effects.

Sedation

Both pregabalin and gabapentin are notorious for their sedative properties. There are a couple of non-medication factors that may exacerbate this dose-dependent adverse effect. Kidney function and age are two risk factors for increasing the risk for sedation and other CNS depressant side effects.

As you can imagine, virtually any medication that is considered a "CNS depressant" or that has this activity can have additive effects to the gabapentinoids. Some of the highest risk CNS depressants include opioids, benzodiazepines, Z-drugs for sleep, TCAs, skeletal muscle relaxants, and older antihistamines.

When assessing a medication list of a patient you want to understand if the patient is already on sedating type medications. If they are, you may look to reduce some of these other agents prior to starting a gabapentinoid. Another strategy is to start with a very low dose. As mentioned above, patients with poor kidney function and advanced age may be at an exacerbated risk for CNS depression. Here's a case scenario where we look at kidney function and the risk of CNS adverse effects accumulating due to multiple medications.

A 78 year old elderly patient had been on a dose of (Neurontin) gabapentin 600 mg three times daily for peripheral neuropathy. She was also on oxycodone and cyclobenzaprine. Over time, the patient's kidney function had been declining and was diagnosed with chronic kidney disease.

The family had begun to notice that the patient was becoming increasingly lethargic and dizzy. The patient had also made the comment that she felt "snowed" from time to time. Meclizine was added as needed to help treat the dizziness and the team decided to monitor the other symptoms at this time. The peripheral neuropathy was well managed with no noted pain stated by the patient.

Because of the decline in kidney function, the previous dose of gabapentin was now inappropriate. This is obvious from the case scenario as the patient is reporting adverse effects. Gabapentin is primarily eliminated from the body through the kidney. The opioid and cyclobenzaprine likely added CNS depressant activity as well. Gabapentin was reduced and the patient's symptoms did resolve. The meclizine added for dizziness was also eventually discontinued as we didn't have any side effects to treat anymore.

Edema

Both gabapentinoids can contribute to edema. We have to be cautious and potentially avoid these agents in patients who have fluid overload. Pay particular attention to patients who may already be taking a diuretic for the purpose of fluid loss. The gabapentinoids can directly oppose the diuretic benefit provided by these medications.

In addition to opposing the beneficial effects of diuretics, we should also recognize if a patient is taking medications that can have additive effects of edema. NSAIDs, calcium channel blockers, and pioglitazone are common examples of medications that can worsen edema. Be really cautious and cognizant of the fact that gabapentinoids can enhance the edema producing effect of these medications.

Angioedema

While angioedema is generally not a substantial concern with gabapentin and pregabalin, there are some case reports that these agents may increase the risk of angioedema in patients already receiving an ACE inhibitor. Unless there is a prior history or something else that may increase the risk of angioedema, this isn't likely a reason or contraindication as to why you would avoid this combination.

Lamotrigine

CNS Depressant

Like many agents that are used to manage bipolar disorder or epilepsy, lamotrigine is considered a CNS depressant. Because of this, it can have additive effects and increase the risk of sedation. I've discussed this in previous sections of this book, so I'll refer you back to the section on opioids.

Reduced Concentrations

Uridine glucuronyl transferase or UGT is an enzyme that likely has some responsibility for deactivating lamotrigine. Phenytoin and carbamazepine have the potential to stimulate the activity of UGT. What this means is that patients will not have as great of response to lamotrigine due to reduced concentrations. If lamotrigine is added to a patient who is already taking phenytoin or carbamazepine, there is a recommendation to get more aggressive with the initial dosing.

On the flipside, we need to be careful about adjusting carbamazepine or phenytoin. If these medications are discontinued, this could send lamotrigine concentrations much higher and increase the risk for adverse effects like cutaneous reactions.

There are a couple of other lower-risk interactions that it would be advisable to be aware of. Acetaminophen and estrogen-based drugs have the potential to reduce concentrations. The extent of this interaction is likely going to depend upon the doses of the medications used, but in the event a patient is experiencing an uptick in seizures or symptoms of bipolar disorder, it would be justified to ensure that these drugs are contributing to the problem.

Increased Concentrations

One really notorious drug interaction with lamotrigine is when it is used in combination with valproic acid. Lamotrigine concentrations can be significantly raised due to this interaction.
One of the most important adverse effects of lamotrigine is rash. As concentrations of lamotrigine rise, the primary risk is for a rash to develop. This can be a life-threatening adverse effect. Be aware of this interaction and recognize that there is a slower dose titration recommendation for lamotrigine if a patient is currently taking valproic acid.

Case Scenario

In this scenario, I take a look at lamotrigine and tramadol amongst other things and why a diagnosis for every medication really matters.

A 71 year old male has been having increasing osteoarthritis pain. He reports pain in his hands, back, and knees. Acetaminophen and

NSAIDs have not seemed to have helped this patient and the provider writes for tramadol 50 mg BID.

Past medical history includes:
- CKD
- Insomnia
- GERD
- Hypertension
- Hyperlipidemia
- Osteoarthritis

Current medications include:
- Amitriptyline 10 mg at bedtime
- Tums 500 mg BID PRN
- Famotidine 20 mg daily
- Aspirin 81 mg daily
- Lamotrigine 250 mg BID
- Norvasc 10 mg daily
- Tramadol 50 mg BID

The first thing that I notice in this scenario is the relatively decent sized dose of lamotrigine. Along with that lamotrigine dose, I notice that the patient doesn't have a diagnosis that would make sense for using this medication. It would concern me that it is being used for seizures and I would be potentially concerned with the tramadol that can lower the seizure threshold. It could definitely be for mood/behavioral disorder, but it is something that needs to be figured out. There is also the potential for a CNS depressant drug interaction between these two.

Having a diagnosis for every medication is so critical. This is likely something that can be obtained through a search of the medical record, but having the diagnosis consistent with the medications can save a lot of time and headache. It can also help us identify concerns much more quickly.

Topiramate

Birth Control
Topiramate has the potential to reduce the concentration of estrogen and progestin containing contraceptives. Here's a case study that demonstrates the risk of this interaction: A 33 year old female has had

an increase in the frequency of migraines over the last few months. She has had about 6 episodes in the last month. These episodes have lasted nearly 24 hours each. The migraines have greatly impacted her quality of life and her triptan use has been escalating.

She was initially placed on propranolol 10 mg twice daily and was titrated upward over a period of a few weeks. She did not like the propranolol and wanted to use a different medication as the propranolol "zonked" her out. The sedative side effect started even at the low dose and got worse as the dose was increased.

She was transitioned to topiramate with relatively good success. Her migraines went down to about 1 per month on average. Three months after initiating the topiramate, she found out that she was pregnant. She had been taking birth control on a regular basis and did not understand how this happened.

The topiramate and birth control interaction is a significant one and in this patient population where pregnancy is a concern and migraines can coexist, it can be a challenge to try to find an agent that prevents migraines and also doesn't cause issues pertaining to pregnancy. Also, remember that valproic acid is usually avoided due to risk to the baby if a patient does become pregnant.

CNS Depressant and Cognition Effects

It is very important to recognize that one of the most frequent adverse effects encountered with topiramate is cognitive impairment. Because of this adverse effect and the brand name of the medication being Topamax, many have given it the nickname of "Dopamax". Like virtually all of the other medications that can be used to manage seizures, topiramate can cause CNS depressant type adverse effects.

Carbonic Anhydrase Inhibitors

Topiramate does have some carbonic anhydrase inhibition activity. In general, other than topiramate, carbonic anhydrase inhibitors are seldom used. The two most common situations I have seen carbonic anhydrase inhibitors used is in the setting of refractory glaucoma and altitude sickness. Acetazolamide is the most commonly used carbonic anhydrase inhibitor.

One big concern with inhibiting carbonic anhydrase is the development of kidney stones. In addition to kidney stones, the risk of metabolic acidosis is a concern. Additive type effects can occur when multiple drugs that inhibit carbonic anhydrase are used together. Carbonic anhydrase inhibitors inhibit the reabsorption of bicarbonate in the kidney. Bicarb exits the body at a higher rate than usual. With the reduction in bicarbonate, the serum pH can go down and thus lead to a state of acidosis. If the pH drops enough, clinical symptoms can develop. In addition to abnormal arterial blood gases, clinical symptoms of metabolic acidosis include rapid breathing, CNS changes like sedation and confusion, and tachycardia.

Hypokalemia

Carbonic anhydrase inhibitors do have a mild diuretic type effect. Because of this, we should be aware that hypokalemia is a risk. This risk is exacerbated by other agents that are also going to cause hypokalemia. Medications that are well known to cause hypokalemia include thiazide and loop diuretics. Keep an extra close eye on electrolytes, specifically potassium, when starting topiramate or any other drug that has carbonic anhydrase inhibiting activity.

Here's a case scenario where a drug with carbonic anhydrase activity led to significant hypokalemia.

A 56 year old male has a history of CHF, diabetes, osteoarthritis, and glaucoma. His current medication list includes:
- Aspirin 81 mg daily
- Losartan 50 mg daily
- Metoprolol 12.5 mg twice daily
- Zaroxolyn 2.5 mg three times per week
- Lasix 80 mg daily
- Tylenol 500-1000 mg TID PRN
- Glipizide XL 5 mg daily
- Xalatan at night

This gentleman had an appointment with his optometrist for further assessment of his glaucoma. Upon returning from the optometrist., he was prescribed oral acetazolamide for glaucoma at 250 mg by mouth twice daily. Prior potassium level a few months before the acetazolamide was 3.5. It was unclear whether the primary physician was unaware of the optometrist appointment or had been notified, but did not recall or anticipate any relevant medication changes. The optometrist did not order any follow up lab work or suggest any when the acetazolamide was ordered for glaucoma.

Acetazolamide is a carbonic anhydrase inhibitor that has a diuretic effect. Topiramate has carbonic anhydrase activity, but to a lesser degree than acetazolamide. This medication, when utilized by itself, would likely have a much lower risk of causing electrolyte abnormalities. When used in combination with other potent diuretics like metolazone and furosemide, the outcome was a little scary. Another factor here was that the potassium was already at the lower end of normal (3.5). When the kidney function and electrolytes were finally rechecked a month or two later after initiation of acetazolamide, the potassium was dangerously low at 2.7.

Levetiracetam

CNS Depressant

Levetiracetam (Keppra) is well known for not having many drug interactions. This is a big advantage of the medication over other medications in this class. In the management of epilepsy, many of the drugs utilized can cause numerous drug interactions. Phenytoin and carbamazepine are two prime examples of epilepsy drugs that have a ton of interactions. While levetiracetam has a low risk for interactions, it is sedating and can have many of the CNS depressant effects that we have discussed before. When assessing sedation and risk for drug interactions, it is ideal if we can reduce other CNS depressant agents that are not being used for a condition as serious as seizure prophylaxis.

Enzyme Inducers

Classic enzyme inducers like carbamazepine and phenytoin have the potential to interact with levetiracetam. It is rare that these agents are used together, but you may see this combination in a patient with refractory seizures. Enzyme inducers are likely to reduce the concentration of levetiracetam. Even though patients may experience lower concentrations of levetiracetam, we are probably unlikely to see an increased risk for seizures as we are adding a seizure medication in phenytoin or carbamazepine.

Donepezil

Anticholinergics

Donepezil is a common agent used to help manage some of the symptoms of Alzheimer's and other types of dementia. Life-threatening drug interactions are usually not a concern with donepezil. However, there are numerous drugs that may blunt the effects of the medication. Any anticholinergic medication that has penetration into the central nervous system is likely to at least partially oppose the potential benefit from donepezil. It is important to avoid these agents in combination with donepezil. Common anticholinergics that I have seen used with donepezil include diphenhydramine, oxybutynin, tolterodine, hydroxyzine, dicyclomine, benztropine, and tricyclic antidepressants.

You may see it flag on drug interaction programs, but the likelihood of respiratory anticholinergics causing any interference with donepezil is slim to none. One should not be hesitant about using long-acting anticholinergic therapy (like tiotropium) or short-acting anticholinergics (like ipratropium) in the setting of COPD or other respiratory distress as indicated.

Bradycardia
Beta-blockers and non-dihydropyridine calcium channel blockers are the most commonly used agents that will suppress the heart rate. We discussed a case scenario of the risk for bradycardia with diltiazem in the calcium channel blocker section.

Additive Effects
There are some less common warnings and precautions that you should be aware of. Some of the precautions may be due to a cumulative effect when other medications are being utilized. In patients who are at risk for GI ulceration due to NSAID use, there is the potential that donepezil and the acetylcholinesterase inhibitors can exacerbate this risk. Minimizing NSAID use, assessing for GI protection, and monitoring for bleed risks are all important factors to consider.

In addition to the GI bleed risk, very rare cases of rhabdomyolysis have been reported as well. As you can imagine, this risk may be exacerbated by the use of statins. Again the chance for rhabdomyolysis is extremely unlikely, but I feel the initiation presents a good time to reassess the goals and values of the patient and their family. In patients who are taking statins, starting a dementia medication presents a good opportunity to go over the risks and benefits of continuing with statin therapy.

Antipsychotics

Much like the interplay between anticholinergics and acetylcholinesterase inhibitors, dopamine agonists and antipsychotics directly oppose each other's effects from a mechanism of action standpoint. Dopamine agonists are going to stimulate dopamine receptors in the brain and antipsychotics are going to reduce dopamine's effect by blocking receptors.

Dopamine agonists are typically going to be used in the setting of RLS, but occasionally you will see them used in Parkinson's disorder. In clinical practice, the likelihood of an antipsychotic medication impacting Parkinson's disease is much more likely than having a negative effect on the management of RLS. This is why recognizing what the dopamine agonist is being used for is important.

If we have a patient with Parkinson's, it is important to recognize the adverse effect profile of different antipsychotics. In general, the first generation, or typical antipsychotics have a much greater potential to cause extrapyramidal symptoms and exacerbate Parkinson's symptoms. The classic example of a first-generation antipsychotic is haloperidol. Because of this disease and drug interaction, we are typically going to avoid the use of all first-generation antipsychotics in favor of the second-generation agents.

When discussing second-generation antipsychotics, they are not all created equal in their impacts on Parkinson's and dopamine agonists. Some second-generation agents like risperidone are more likely to negatively impact Parkinson's. Clozapine, pimavanserin, and quetiapine are all considered second-generation agents that have a better adverse effect profile to be used in Parkinson's. In clinical practice from a cost-effectiveness and safety perspective, quetiapine is the most commonly used agent that I have seen used in this situation.

Hypotension

Dopamine agonists have the potential to lower blood pressure. When discussing hypertension we talked about this risk. For dopamine agonists, hypotension is a dose-dependent effect meaning that if you have a patient on a higher dose, that patient is more likely to experience this adverse effect. Whether the antihypertensive effect is planned or not, keep an eye out for other drugs that drop blood pressure. We can also assess patients by checking orthostatic blood pressure readings, asking about dizziness with position changes, and also inquiring about the frequency and timing of falls.

CYP1A2

Inhibitors of CYP1A2 can raise the concentration of ropinirole and increase the potential for adverse effects. Classic examples of drugs that can inhibit CYP1A2 include fluvoxamine and ciprofloxacin. If this is a concern, a simple reduction in the dose of the ropinirole would be appropriate. Interestingly, smoking cigarettes can actually induce CYP1A2 which may lead to lower concentrations of ropinirole. Alternatively, pramipexole does avoid the CYP1A2 pathway, so if this is a concern, a transition to this dopamine agonist could be considered.

Sumatriptan

Serotonin Syndrome

Triptans have been associated with serotonin syndrome. The overwhelming majority of agents used in the management of depression have some amount of activity on serotonin receptors. Using sumatriptan for migraines in a patient taking an SSRI is commonly done without much risk for issues. However, it may be advisable to review patient history, the severity of migraine, and the intensity of antidepressant therapy prior to initiating a triptan. I have more reservations about using a triptan in a patient on a high dose SSRI versus those taking a low dose (i.e. fluoxetine 80 mg daily versus 20 mg daily).

Contraindicated Drug Interactions

I think it is probably pretty obvious, but for completeness sake, sumatriptan should not be used in combination with any other triptan. Also, recall that drugs like dihydroergotamine and other ergot derivatives should not be used in combination with triptans. In addition to this, MAOIs and drugs with MAOI activity should not be used in combination with the triptans. Common drugs with MAOI activity that I have seen used in clinical practice include tranylcypromine, phenelzine, and linezolid.

Cardiovascular Medications

There are some risks involving the cardiovascular system that have been rarely encountered with the use of triptans. Elevations in blood pressure, myocardial infarction, and stroke have all been reported with these agents. Again, this risk is very rare. I will take a look at a patient's medication list when triptans are being used. If you notice a patient is taking numerous medications indicating a significant cardiovascular history, you might want to stop and reassess the risk versus benefits of triptan therapy and consider what our alternatives might include. When reviewing a medication list for risk of cardiovascular events, I look for items like dual antiplatelet therapy, antihypertensives, statin use, nitrates, indicators of smoking, and diabetes. If you see a lot of these concerns in their medication list or medical history, you might have a little more cause for concern when using a triptan.

Valproic Acid

Seizure Risk

When using valproic acid, it is critical to know what the indication is. I've seen this drug be used for seizures, bipolar disorder, migraines, aggressive behaviors in dementia, and many more indications. I'm definitely more cautious when it comes to drug interactions when it is specifically being used for seizures. Drugs that can reduce concentrations and drugs that lower the seizure threshold are big concerns. Carbapenems, tramadol, and bupropion are all medications that may increase the risk for seizures and we should avoid using these if possible in a patient that has a history of seizures and is being managed with valproic acid.

Rifampin, barbiturates, carbamazepine, and phenytoin are all potential enzyme inducers that can increase the metabolism of valproic acid. Again, if it is being used for epilepsy, we have to be aware that we may put our patients at higher risk for a seizure.

Protein Binding

There are drugs that can alter the protein binding of valproic acid. Drugs compete with valproic acid for binding sites on protein in the blood. When this happens, it can increase the free fraction of valproic acid. When more drug is freely circulating in the bloodstream, it is able to produce its physiologic effects. Phenytoin is a classic example of a medication that is highly protein-bound. When phenytoin is added, it can essentially kick valproic acid off of protein in the blood and increase the risk for toxicity. This is a two-way street and valproic acid can compete against phenytoin leading to a higher free fraction of phenytoin in the blood. With this interaction specifically, remember that phenytoin can lower concentrations of valproic acid by enzyme induction. In clinical practice, this makes this interaction incredibly difficult to predict.

Lamotrigine

I discussed the valproic acid and lamotrigine interaction under the lamotrigine section. Valproic acid increases the risk for lamotrigine induced toxicity and Stevens-Johnson syndrome.

Lorazepam

I would technically classify valproic acid as having CNS depressant type activity so any of the previously mentioned interactions on CNS depressants should be monitored for. Assessing for excessive sedation is important in patients taking more than one sedating agent together.

Lorazepam is a little bit special. Being a part of the benzodiazepine class, it is without a doubt a drug that will cause CNS depression. In addition to this adverse effect, valproic acid has the potential to increase the serum concentration. Valproic acid likely interferes with the UGT enzymes that breakdown lorazepam. Because of this, concentrations of lorazepam can rise and toxicity may be more likely to occur.

Liver Toxicity

Valproic acid has a boxed warning for liver toxicity. This is something that I remember when looking through a medication list. I specifically pay attention to other medications that may be liver toxic and have additive effects to the liver toxic nature of valproic acid. Many of the other antiepileptic agents like carbamazepine and phenytoin carry this risk. Two other commonly used agents with warnings on liver toxicity include amiodarone and methotrexate. Also, recall that isoniazid for tuberculosis carries this risk. Avoidance of using two or more liver toxic agents together is ideal. Certainly, we need to monitor liver function in patients taking valproic acid or any of these agents mentioned.

Enzyme Induction – CYP3A4

Much like rifampin and carbamazepine, phenytoin is a potent inducer of CYP3A4. The clinical impact of using phenytoin is real and something that should not be taken lightly. When I see it being used, it is definitely one of those medications that I look up every medication and run a drug interaction screen.

Common CYP3A4 interactions include effects on medications like diltiazem, verapamil, apixaban, rivaroxaban, atorvastatin, amiodarone, simvastatin, and warfarin. In the overwhelming majority of situations, adding phenytoin to a patient's regimen will be likely to cause reduced concentrations.

P-glycoprotein Induction

Much like rifampin and carbamazepine, phenytoin has the ability to induce P-glycoprotein. The risk for subtherapeutic concentrations with apixaban and rivaroxaban exist with phenytoin just as they do with rifampin and carbamazepine.

Albumin Displacement

Phenytoin is strongly protein-bound and can displace other drugs or can be displaced by other medications. Valproic acid and warfarin are two examples that come to mind. When phenytoin is displaced from serum protein like albumin, the consequence is a higher free fraction of drug. When there is a higher free fraction, there is more drug freely available to produce physiological effects.

In addition to the displacement drug interactions above, alterations in albumin levels can impact the clinical effects of phenytoin. When albumin levels are higher (or normal) there is more albumin available to "stick" to phenytoin. When albumin levels go lower, there is less albumin for the phenytoin to bind to. When albumin is low, what this leads to is a significantly higher amount of free phenytoin which can exert its activity in the body.

The most common scenario I've seen low albumin in is in malnourished patients. You may see a higher likelihood of phenytoin toxicity even at "normal" total blood concentrations in a patient who has low albumin.

There are a few ways to monitor this. The first step is to monitor for signs/symptoms of toxicity or seizures if that is the indication we are using phenytoin for. Checking albumin levels can also be helpful to assess any trends that may alter the free fraction of phenytoin. Assessing a "free" phenytoin level is an appropriate action to take as well if there is a concern that protein binding is skewing the total phenytoin levels. There is also a corrected phenytoin level equation that can be of some assistance. It is primarily based upon the albumin level. All monitoring tools should be used hand in hand with sound clinical monitoring.

Vitamin D Deficiency

In the Vitamin D section, we discussed a case scenario where phenytoin caused vitamin D deficiency. It is important to remember that patients who take phenytoin may be at risk of phenytoin causing induction of vitamin D metabolism. Being aware of this risk and paying attention to the risk for fractures and subtherapeutic vitamin D levels is very important.

Memantine

Carbonic Anhydrase Inhibitors

Memantine has a relatively low risk for drug interactions. I discussed carbonic anhydrase inhibitors in a little more detail when I discussed topiramate, but what I didn't mention is that drugs with this activity can raise the concentrations of memantine. Pay attention to signs and symptoms of memantine adverse effects. Topiramate, acetazolamide, and zonisamide are the most commonly used agents I've seen in clinical practice that have carbonic anhydrase inhibition activity. Carbonic anhydrase inhibitors used for glaucoma for eye administration are generally not going to have enough systemic absorption to cause any issues with memantine.

Trimethoprim

Memantine and trimethoprim may increase each other's concentrations. Assess for signs and symptoms of toxicity from either agent. Both of these agents rely heavily on renal elimination and they are likely to compete with each other for organic cation transporters in the kidney. By competing with each other for this transporter, less of each drug will be transported out of the body.

Anticholinergics

While anticholinergics do not directly oppose the beneficial effects of memantine from a mechanistic standpoint, they can oppose the cognitive effects we are trying to promote. Because of the adverse effect of cognitive impairment and confusion that anticholinergics can cause, they can oppose the potential benefits from any medication used specifically for dementia. It is critical to try to minimize the anticholinergic burden in any patient with dementia whether they are treated with medications or not.

Meclizine

Anticholinergic/Antihistamine Activity

Meclizine has a variety of different adverse effects and a lot of them can be determined by the mechanism of action. While it can have a lot of different drug interactions due to antihistamine and anticholinergic activity, meclizine doses are usually pretty low and infrequent as the medication is typically only used as needed for motion sickness and vertigo symptoms. Meclizine has anticholinergic activity and can contribute to anticholinergic burden. We have discussed this extensively in the antihistamine portion of the book and will refer to that section for further information.

CNS Depressant

Any antihistamine is sedating by nature and can exacerbate the sedating effect of many other agents. In the setting of vertigo, this may be advantageous to help a patient rest through an episode. With the low doses typically utilized, the risk for excessive CNS sedation is pretty low unless escalation in other CNS depressant medications accompanies the use of meclizine.

Carbidopa/Levodopa

Dopamine Antagonism

I briefly mentioned the interplay between dopamine agonists and dopamine antagonists when I discussed the use of ropinirole. Carbidopa/levodopa is essentially a replacement of dopamine in the brain. There are numerous medications that can blunt the beneficial effects of levodopa in Parkinson's disorder. Here's a case scenario that demonstrates the prescribing cascade, and the risk of dopamine

185

antagonism in a patient needing levodopa replacement for management of their Parkinson's disease.

An 82 year old male has a medical history of osteoarthritis, diabetes, BPH, gastroparesis and Parkinson's disease. He is complaining of nausea and stomach upset after meals. Current medications include:

- Sinemet 25/100 mg 2 tablets three times daily
- Requip 0.5 mg BID
- Protonix 40 mg once daily
- Aspirin 81 mg daily
- Oxybutynin 5 mg TID
- Diphenhydramine 50 mg HS
- Metformin 500 mg BID
- Acetaminophen 500 mg PRN
- Atorvastatin 10 mg daily
- Senna S 1 BID

This is a situation set up for the classic prescribing cascade. We have a new or exacerbated symptom of possible gastroparesis. The most common medication I see used in the setting of gastroparesis is metoclopramide and that is what the primary provider would like to prescribe. The major issue with metoclopramide is that it does block dopamine receptors and could exacerbate this gentleman's Parkinson's disease.

What I would like to address first is the use of the anticholinergics. Remember that anticholinergics can slow down the GI tract and possibly contribute to constipation and/or gastroparesis. Identifying why this patient is using diphenhydramine (likely for insomnia) and finding an alternative would be an appropriate consideration. Also looking at BPH and how/why this patient is on the oxybutynin would be another important aspect in trying to rule out drug-induced gastroparesis.

If we can minimize the anticholinergic burden, we may be able to avoid the use of metoclopramide. Avoiding metoclopramide would help us sidestep the potential for it to exacerbate Parkinson's and oppose the beneficial effects of levodopa.

Hypotension

As we have discussed, several agents can lower blood pressure and have additive effects on one another. Carbidopa/levodopa falls within the category of agents that can contribute to orthostasis. The big challenge with the use of carbidopa/levodopa is that Parkinson's patients are already at risk for falls due to their movement disorder. In addition, Parkinson's disease alone can increase the risk of orthostatic hypotension without the help of medications. Paying attention to blood pressure and fall risk is huge. If the patient's movement symptoms are well controlled, and the blood pressure is concerningly low, we should look at reducing other blood pressure-lowering agents first. If they are not on any other blood pressure-lowering medications, then reducing the dose of carbidopa/levodopa may be considered. We would want to take a good hard assessment as to when symptoms of low blood pressure or falls are happening and make further determinations from there as to the next steps.

Here's a real-life scenario and how I would approach it.

An 86 year old male is having a difficult time with weakness and falls. With weakness and falls, we always need to take a good hard look at blood pressure to make sure we aren't causing drug-induced orthostasis. There are also times when the family feels like he is very sleepy. He also had mild cognition problems. His latest vital signs were BP = 102/76 with a drop to 72/54 when an orthostatic reading was checked. His pulse is 62 beats per minute. His current medications include;

- Aspirin 81 mg daily
- Tamsulosin 0.4 mg daily
- Sinemet 25/100 TID
- Requip 1 mg TID
- Norvasc 2.5 mg daily
- Gabapentin 800 mg four times daily
- Famotidine 20 mg daily
- Acetaminophen 500 mg QID PRN
- Latanoprost 1 gtt in the left eye at bedtime

Blood pressure is obviously well within the goal and the amlodipine should likely be discontinued in this scenario. We'd like to keep the dose of carbidopa/levodopa the same if symptoms of Parkinson's are well controlled.

While gabapentin is not well-known for causing low blood pressure, it can certainly be associated with falls. This is an extremely high dose in an 86 year old and should be considered for reduction.

If orthostasis and other symptoms continue despite changes in the Norvasc and gabapentin, the next two drugs that should be looked at are tamsulosin, Sinemet, and ropinirole. With a likely diagnosis of Parkinson's, changing the Parkinson's medications can be a significant challenge and he is at a starting dose of the Sinemet, but the Requip dose is a fairly decent one.

Binding Interactions

Carbidopa/levodopa can be a very tricky drug. If the dose is too high, the patient can experience side effects like nausea, vomiting, hallucination, low blood pressure, and dyskinesia. If the dose is too low, the signs of Parkinson's disorder can take over. Binding interactions can play a role in altering those concentrations and if a patient who was previously well-controlled presents with escalating Parkinson's symptoms, the possibility for a binding interaction should be considered.

Oral iron products are likely going to be the most common medication that can impact concentrations of levodopa. Ensure that your patient actually needs long term iron. If iron is necessary, we reduce the risk by attempting to separate the timing of administration. Try to administer iron a couple hours before or after the carbidopa/levodopa.

It is important to assess the patient clinically. They may present to you taking both iron and carbidopa/levodopa and have no concerns with their Parkinson's symptoms. If this is the case, it would be prudent to recognize the interaction, but assume that their dose is adjusted accordingly to the interaction. In the event iron is ever discontinued, it would be important to assess for signs of carbidopa/levodopa toxicity.

Carbamazepine

Carbamazepine Can Interact With Carbamazepine?

Yes, you are reading that correctly. In one of the most unique twists with drug interactions, carbamazepine can actually stimulate the metabolism of itself. While this is really intriguing, what you really want to know is what to do with this clinically?

Here's the easy answer to this question...it depends. I think I've stressed plenty of times throughout the book already, but you have to know what you are treating. With carbamazepine, we typically monitor and shoot for target levels in patients with epilepsy or bipolar disorder. In patients with trigeminal neuralgia, we usually treat to symptom relief and only assess levels if trying to rule out toxicity.

Back to why this matters. In patients that we are trying to maintain steady levels, these levels can vary significantly within the first few weeks and up to a month or two following initiation because of enzyme induction. Levels can be initially higher and once autoinduction ramps up, they may drop significantly. Clinical monitoring as well as checking levels is important upon initiation until a patient's level is deemed stable. In situations where we are not shooting for a target level, we may only do this to monitor for risk of toxicity versus targeting a goal for therapeutic benefit.

Enzyme Induction

Whenever I see an order for carbamazepine, I have alarms going off in my head. Carbamazepine is an enzyme inducer. The primary cause of the majority of drug interactions is due to the induction of CYP3A4. P-glycoprotein induction may also play a significant role in some drug interactions. In most situations, the carbamazepine will reduce concentrations of other medications.

Anticoagulants like apixaban, rivaroxaban, warfarin, and dabigatran can all have their concentrations reduced. The result of this can be catastrophic by increasing the risk of stroke. Certain antipsychotics can have their effectiveness reduced. Many HIV medications will also interact with carbamazepine. Antibiotics and many antidepressants can have significant interactions with carbamazepine. There are simply too many drug interactions to list with this drug. I cannot overstate this. I also do not have them all memorized. When I have a patient on carbamazepine, I run a drug interaction profile to ensure the patient is not taking other medications that interact with it. Rather than attempt to memorize all the potential interactions, this is what I would recommend you do as well.

CYP1A2 Induction

Carbamazepine can be responsible for the induction of CYP1A2 as well. This is generally considered to be a much smaller impact than the CYP3A4 induction. Antipsychotics like clozapine and olanzapine can have their concentrations reduced on account of the interaction with carbamazepine.

Hyponatremia

Drug-induced SIADH is a real possibility with carbamazepine. Because of this, if the patient is experiencing any symptoms of hyponatremia like sedation, confusion, nausea, vomiting, or weakness, these drugs should be reassessed. When carbamazepine is used with other agents that may cause hyponatremia, this risk is amplified. The use of diuretics like hydrochlorothiazide or chlorthalidone may increase this risk. In addition, other medications that have been associated with SIADH may have a compounding type effect.

The urgency of dealing with this drug interaction is going to be largely dependent upon the severity of hyponatremia. If a patient is displaying CNS symptoms and their sodium level is in the 120's or less, these drugs will likely have to be stopped unless there is another identifiable cause. If carbamazepine is for seizures, this obviously gets a lot trickier. If the patient has mild hyponatremia, such as a level in the low 130's mEq/L and is not displaying symptoms, some clinicians may decide to continue to monitor sodium levels and leave the medications in place. Weighing the risk of complications from hyponatremia compared to the benefit of drug therapy is critical. If other options are available that are less likely to cause hyponatremia, switching medications seems like the best option.

Oxcarbazepine

Carbamazepine's Cousin

Oxcarbazepine is definitely an improvement over carbamazepine when we look specifically at drug interactions. It is not used very often, but I wanted to mention it because of this fact. Oxcarbazepine is not considered to carry as large of a CYP3A4 induction risk that carbamazepine has. Combining oxcarbazepine is not recommended with many HIV medications like dolutegravir, tenofovir alafenamide, or elvitegravir. This is primarily due to a reduction in concentrations which could lead to treatment failure and risk for developing resistance.

Again, I'd encourage you to look up interactions if you see oxcarbazepine being utilized. One last possible enzyme induction interaction I wanted to mention specifically was the risk with birth control. Because so many patients take oral contraceptives, we must recognize that both carbamazepine and oxcarbazepine can reduce their effectiveness. Patients need to be aware of this and seek alternative methods for preventing pregnancy.

Oxcarbazepine, like carbamazepine, still carries the risk for SIADH and hyponatremia. It is important to recognize agents that may have hyponatremia inducing effects.

Serotonin Syndrome Risk

There are a large number of medications that can contribute to the risk of serotonin syndrome. The SSRIs are usually the first class of medication I think of as being able to contribute to this risk. Individual drug members of the SSRI class include citalopram, escitalopram, fluoxetine, paroxetine, sertraline, fluvoxamine, vilazodone, and vortioxetine.

In addition to the SSRIs, other classes of medications that can increase the risk of serotonin syndrome include, SNRIs, TCAs, MAOIs, triptans, amphetamines, antipsychotics, and 5HT3 antagonists. Other relatively common individual drugs that can raise the risk of serotonin syndrome include linezolid, tramadol, buspirone, metoclopramide, lithium, and cyclobenzaprine. MAOIs and drugs with significant MAOI activity should be avoided in combination with SSRIs. There may be situations of a cross-taper to another class, but in general, TCA, SNRI and SSRI combinations are avoided. Often times many of the other agents will be used in combination with an SSRI with the clinician having to evaluate the risk of serotonin syndrome versus the potential benefit that the patient might be getting from the medication that is going to be initiated.

While the risk for serotonin syndrome is absolutely real, I think many clinicians struggle with how seriously to take this drug interaction. To give you some context, I've only encountered a couple of case reports of serotonin syndrome throughout my 10+ year career. While extremely rare, because of the seriousness of this adverse effect, I do not think it should be overlooked. Here's a classic example of a combination that is often seen in practice that can raise the risk of serotonin syndrome.

A 64 year old female is taking sertraline 25 mg daily and tramadol 50 mg as needed for back pain. She reports that she probably only uses the tramadol one or two times per week on average. Dispensing records back up her utilization pattern for the tramadol. We should never exclude anything if a patient presents with symptoms of a condition like serotonin syndrome, but if I have a patient on sertraline 25 mg daily and is taking a PRN tramadol 50 mg once or twice a week this isn't going to be a big concern to me. In the absence of symptoms, serotonin syndrome is likely not going to be the first thing on my radar, to say the least.

Compare the previously mentioned example to a patient on sertraline 200 mg daily and venlafaxine 300 mg daily. My concern for serotonin syndrome is obviously much greater and we would need to thoroughly investigate why those high doses and why this combination is being used. The combination would also lead you to ask the question if we've had to ramp up to these doses on both medications, have they really been effective? I would also consider it inappropriate to use an SSRI in combination with an SNRI. Given the venlafaxine and sertraline combination, my level of concern for serotonin syndrome risk would be much higher than a patient simply on a low dose SSRI and who takes an occasional tramadol.

Here's one last case example in trying to differentiate whether a patient may be presenting with serotonin syndrome versus adverse effects.

An 88 y/o female presents to your care. She's had some difficulty with pain management. She was on scheduled Tylenol (acetaminophen) 1,000 mg twice daily as well as Ultram (tramadol) 50 mg every 6 hours as needed. She had brought up the complaint about her osteoarthritis to her physician. She was prescribed tramadol 100 mg four times daily scheduled. When I had spoken with the caregivers, they had been doing some research and were significantly concerned about serotonin syndrome due to increased confusion, a general decline in her condition and worsening mental status. In addition to the newly increased tramadol, this patient was on citalopram 20 mg daily.

In assessing the patient from a clinical perspective, there were no other symptoms of serotonin syndrome (like tachycardia, elevated temperature, etc.) besides the change in cognition. Serotonin syndrome is very serious, but the cause of the symptoms was likely from an inappropriately aggressive increase in the tramadol. Upon discussion with caregivers, she was only taking the PRN Ultram one or two times daily on average. The increase from 50-100 mg of tramadol per day to 400 mg per day was simply too aggressive in this case and this was the cause of the adverse effects. Another key point is that the maximum recommended daily dose for tramadol is 300 mg for the elderly. Adverse effects improved with a reduction in the tramadol to 50 mg three times daily.

Antiplatelet Activity

SSRIs have the potential to interfere with platelet activity. The clinical impact of this still remains a little murky and may vary based upon the dose and the specific SSRI that is being used. I did spend some time discussing this risk in the aspirin and NSAID section, but I wanted to lay out a scenario and give you my thoughts on how to handle a clinical situation. I want to breakdown a situation where a 77 year old female patient on citalopram 20 mg daily is being placed on apixaban for atrial fibrillation. Here are a few thoughts on what I think about with this combination and the potential risk for bleeding.

- My first step is to do an assessment of past bleed history. Have they had a GI bleed or other type of bleed in the past? Are they taking any other medications that could exacerbate this risk?
- Are they taking any other over-the-counter medications that we don't know about that could also increase risk? The most common OTCs would include traditional NSAIDs or aspirin.
- If both medications are indicated and appropriate, is GI protection with a PPI or other agent necessary? Depending upon the risk for GI bleed, this may be an appropriate indication for a long term PPI.
- Monitoring of labs like hemoglobin and platelets would be a strong consideration in this case. You're likely going to assess these factors with the use of apixaban anyway, but having the citalopram on board makes it slightly more important.
- What doses are we at for each agent? The platelet inhibition effect from SSRIs is dose-dependent. The higher the dose, the more likely you will have platelet inhibition.
- Can we select an alternative antidepressant? This may or may not be appropriate given the circumstances, but it is a very pertinent question to ask. A drug like bupropion would likely have a lower risk for antiplatelet activity and potentially lower risk of inducing bleeding.
- Monitor and educate. Letting patients know that there could be an increased risk of bleeding in using these two medications together is always a good idea as patients can help monitor for signs and symptoms of bruising or bleeding. This is probably the course of action most providers will take in managing this interaction, but there are numerous factors that could alter that assessment

QTc Prolongation

All of the SSRIs have been associated with QTc prolongation. QTc prolongation is a cumulative effect. To be clinically significant, a patient typically has to have risk factors for QTc prolongation and/or be taking other medications that increase the risk. Within the class of the SSRIs, some agents are considered higher risk than others. In general, citalopram has the most evidence as being problematic. Escitalopram is structurally very close to citalopram and carries some risk as well. Other agents in this class are associated with QTc prolongation, but probably to a lesser extent than citalopram or escitalopram.

How does this play out clinically? In a patient who is deemed to have a low risk for QTc prolongation, using citalopram versus sertraline probably isn't a concern with regards to the cardiac implications. If you have a patient where QTc prolongation is an issue or they are taking a drug like amiodarone, you'll likely want to avoid citalopram and possibly escitalopram in favor of another SSRI like sertraline or fluoxetine.

Opposition of Sexual Dysfunction Medications

SSRIs are a notorious cause of medication-induced sexual dysfunction. Here's a case scenario where this adverse effect can directly oppose the benefit we are trying to provide with the use of sildenafil.

A 47 year old male is concerned that his drugs are causing medication-induced sexual dysfunction. His primary provider has asked you to review his medications. What would I look at here?
- Amlodipine 5 mg daily
- Metoprolol 25 mg twice daily
- Fluoxetine 80 mg daily
- Bupropion 150 mg daily
- Lansoprazole 15 mg once daily
- Tums as needed
- Sildenafil 100 mg as needed for sexual dysfunction
- Aspirin 81 mg daily
- Metformin 500 mg twice daily

When I first look at a medication list, I try to pull out really common medications that I am aware of that could cause medication-induced sexual dysfunction. I like to come up with solutions to problems and this one likely does present a challenge.

The fluoxetine is also at a substantially high dose. This makes me believe that the patient has significant mental health concerns. He is also taking the bupropion. There is potential to try to increase the bupropion dose and with that maybe we could reduce the fluoxetine if it is being used for something like depression. Avoiding or reducing the fluoxetine may help us to avoid the potential adverse effect of sexual dysfunction.

There are blood pressure medications that can cause drug-induced sexual dysfunction. The second medication that I would look at is the metoprolol. If being used simply for hypertension without any other compelling indications like previous MI, atrial fibrillation, etc. this is a medication we could possibly change. Amlodipine is a much better medication as far as its risk in contributing to medication-induced sexual dysfunction. Increasing this dose would likely not cause further issues if the metoprolol could be reduced and/or discontinued.

When I think of sexual dysfunction and am able to work with patients on a problem like this, I also do my best to remind them that their medical conditions can cause these problems. In this situation, it would be an important point to remind the patient that his hypertension and diabetes could contribute to this problem. Any lifestyle changes he would be willing to make could help improve his sexual dysfunction.

SIADH

In an example of the prescribing cascade, I had a resident at a nursing home that was prescribed Lexapro for depressive and anxiety type symptoms. A few weeks after starting this medication, the resident had worsening confusion, change in cognition, and was getting physically and verbally aggressive with staff. It was apparent that something was going on.

Seroquel an antipsychotic was ordered to try to help with the delirium and aggressive type symptoms. Lexapro was continued for a few more days, and labs were ordered to try to decipher what was the cause of the change in status. Labs revealed that the resident had hyponatremia (low sodium) which can be caused by Lexapro. Lexapro was discontinued, the low sodium resolved and the resident was doing better. I can't stress enough the importance of trying to avoid the use of other medications (i.e. Seroquel in this case) to treat side effects of other medications!

Sertraline

I want to cover the individual SSRIs as there are some differences in their drug interaction profiles. Sertraline is considered the most serotonergic agent in relation to gut activity and there are a couple of situations that you should remember when it comes to drug interactions. Sertraline is often coined as "Squirtraline" for its potential to contribute to diarrhea. Pay attention to other medications that may exacerbate this adverse effect. Many chemotherapy agents, antibiotics, metformin, and colchicine are examples of agents with a relatively high incidence of diarrhea.

In addition, patients with preexisting GI diseases like IBS or IBD are at risk for diarrhea. In a patient with predominant symptoms of diarrhea, we would likely want to avoid sertraline as it could have opposite effects of some of the medications we may be using to try to manage diarrhea from the GI disease.

Paroxetine

Paroxetine has the greatest amount of anticholinergic activity of all of the SSRIs. Because of this fact, it can compound the problem of anticholinergic burden in patients taking other anticholinergic medications. If other SSRIs have not been tried, the use of paroxetine is generally discouraged in the elderly.

In addition to having anticholinergic activity, it is also well known for inhibiting CYP2D6. Codeine, tramadol, aripiprazole, atomoxetine, bupropion, and metoclopramide are a few common examples of medications that may be affected by CYP2D6 inhibition. A drug interaction that is an absolute contraindication is tamoxifen. Here's a case scenario regarding this interaction.

A 56 year old female has been having increased depressive symptoms and was placed on paroxetine 20 mg daily. Her other medications include:
- Aspirin 81 mg daily
- Tamoxifen 20 mg daily
- Lansoprazole 30 mg daily
- Docusate 100 mg daily
- Ibuprofen 400 mg as needed

- Vitamin D 1000 units daily

When reviewing a drug interaction, the first thing I look at is what is going to be the result of this interaction. In the case of paroxetine interacting with tamoxifen, the end result will potentially be a reduced tamoxifen concentration. In someone using tamoxifen for breast cancer, this is obviously a significant concern.

Another important question is how does this interaction happen. Tamoxifen is considered a prodrug. A prodrug gets converted by the body (through enzymes) to an active form (or more active form). In this case, that enzyme is CYP2D6. CYP2D6 is inhibited by paroxetine. Giving paroxetine to a patient who is taking tamoxifen will, therefore, block the conversion of tamoxifen to the more active form that provides the benefit to the patient.

With some interactions (particularly many binding interactions), we can alter the timing of doses and still keep the patient on the medications that are desired. Unfortunately, in this case, the most appropriate action would be to identify an alternative antidepressant. You must remember however that many other antidepressants can inhibit 2D6 as well. Fluoxetine and bupropion are two more examples that can impact CYP2D6.

One of the most challenging aspects of drug interactions is that you can often find conflicting evidence. If you do a literature search on this, you will find reports of this tamoxifen paroxetine interaction having no impact. However, it is always important to play it on the safe side if other alternatives exist.

Citalopram

QTc prolongation is one of the bigger risks that is specifically associated with citalopram. Paying attention to risk factors, elevated baseline QTc interval and concomitant medications that may prolong the QT interval is very important in assessing this effect. We've already discussed many of the drugs that can impact the QT interval under the amiodarone section.

Escitalopram

Other than citalopram, QTc prolongation is likely a more significant concern with escitalopram than any other SSRI. Similar to citalopram, pay attention to other medications and risk factors for QTc prolongation. Similar to citalopram, inhibition of CYP2C19 can significantly raise the concentrations of escitalopram.

Fluoxetine

Much like paroxetine, fluoxetine can inhibit CYP2D6 to a significant extent. It will have a very similar drug interaction profile to paroxetine.

Here's a case scenario involving the Prozac Wellbutrin interaction. A 64 year old male has severe depression. He is currently on Remeron 15 mg once daily, Prozac 80 mg once daily, and Abilify 10 mg once daily. He has been tried on just about every other SSRI and SNRI without any benefit. He is still reporting that he would like something in addition to his current regimen.

Abilify was tried at a higher dose, but the patient experienced troublesome tremors and other extrapyramidal symptoms. Remeron was also tried at higher doses and the patient reported that he had nightmares and abnormal dreams on the 30 mg dose. Tri-cyclic antidepressants have also been tried in the past with no benefit. The patient cannot recall if he has been on Wellbutrin and the psychiatrist working with him did not see any contraindications to adding it.

A prescription is written for Wellbutrin XL 150 mg once daily for 7 days and increase to 300 mg once daily after that.

At about week 2, the patient is reporting significant anxiety and insomnia. Upon assessment, he is also having some tachycardia and has a slightly elevated temperature. He believes that it is likely from the addition of the Wellbutrin. The patient is likely correct in the situation in that these are probably side effects of medication, but you certainly could make an argument that the side effects may be from the Prozac.

The Prozac Wellbutrin interaction is one to put in your storage bank. Wellbutrin is an inhibitor of CYP2D6 and could potentially lead to increased concentrations of Prozac. If we dig a little deeper and look at this from a clinical perspective, the patient may be beginning to display mild signs and symptoms of serotonin syndrome.

I see situations similar to this when it comes to drug interactions and often times what puts some patients over the top and into the danger zone is the dosing of the medication. This particular patient was already on a high dose of the Prozac and the Wellbutrin was escalated to a decent dose as well. Having a patient on this high of a dose of Prozac probably enhanced the concentrations of the drug dramatically. When assessing interactions like this, (hopefully prior to initiating medication), you have got to look at the relative doses and consider them prior to starting therapy.

In this Prozac Wellbutrin interaction scenario, the very high dose of Prozac probably led to this interaction being a very significant one for the patient.

Fluvoxamine

While the likelihood of seeing fluvoxamine used in clinical practice is low, I did want to include it because there are so many drug interactions associated with its use.

Fluvoxamine can inhibit CYP1A2, CYP2C19, and CYP3A4. Because of the ability to inhibit all of these three enzymes, the risk for drug interactions is high with the use of fluvoxamine. We've discussed several medications throughout the book that are impacted by these enzymes. This is another drug that I personally do not have all of these interactions memorized and I would strongly encourage you to run this drug through an interaction screen when starting new medications or starting fluvoxamine itself.

I had a resident in a nursing home who had an extensive psych history including episodes of physical aggression and schizophrenia. They also would be extremely obsessive over various different things from time to time. There were followed closely by psychiatry. This patient was receiving a dose of Zyprexa (olanzapine) of 15 mg at bedtime. To help with the obsessive/compulsive disorder (OCD) the psychiatrist ordered Luvox (fluvoxamine). Fluvoxamine is an SSRI but is rarely used due to the potential for multiple drug interactions. Within a few days upon initiation of the Luvox, the patient was extremely lethargic and had a couple of falls. The most likely cause of this was an interaction where Luvox can significantly increase the blood levels of Zyprexa, leading to potential toxicity. If you ever see an order for Luvox, you must look for drug interactions!

Benzodiazepines

CNS Depressant

Benzodiazepines are a classic example of a medication that can cause sedation, fatigue and a general central nervous system depressant effect. Common examples of benzodiazepines include alprazolam, clonazepam, lorazepam, diazepam, and temazepam. We've discussed this at length in the opioid section, but I wanted to make sure to include it here as these drugs can be very sedating. In addition, the risk for respiratory depression, when used in combination with opioids, is a significant concern.

A good way I recall the adverse effect profile of benzodiazepines is to compare it to alcohol. It has a lot of similarities. Sedation, ataxia, fall risk, slurred speech, cognitive impairment can all occur as the dose of benzodiazepines escalate. We have to be careful about using alcohol with benzodiazepines. It is best to avoid this combination altogether to avoid the risk of cumulative effects.

Benzodiazepines can often be used for their sedative effects. I've encountered numerous patients taking benzodiazepines for insomnia. It is very important to remember to look for drugs that may oppose the beneficial action of sedation. Here's a case example:

A 66 year old male patient who was rehabbing a knee replacement, was also having difficulty sleeping. Pain was pretty well managed and eventually determined not to be a significant factor in this case. I had discussed the case with nursing, and they stated that he was up all day and all night and did have some anxiety, but he was more concerned that he couldn't sleep. Nursing was questioning if we could try some lorazepam to help with this problem. I said I'd take a look and see what I could figure out. I did not anticipate when reviewing the medication list that the patient would be on a stimulant type medication.

This patient was taking Provigil (modafinil) for an unknown reason. I suspect it was maybe to help stimulate energy for rehab as I have seen this off label a couple of different times. Always, always, always look for a drug-related reason for the symptoms a patient is experiencing! The modafinil was discontinued and sleep patterns improved. We also avoided the unnecessary use of Ativan to treat side effects that the modafinil was causing.

CYP3A4 Effects

CYP3A4 is a critical enzyme for the breakdown of alprazolam. Because of this pharmacokinetic fact, numerous drugs can impact the concentration of alprazolam. Azole antifungals, clarithromycin, grapefruit juice, verapamil, diltiazem, and other agents that inhibit

CYP3A4 will be likely to cause elevations in alprazolam concentrations. Be aware that patients who present with adverse effects from a stable dose of alprazolam may have encountered a drug interaction.

On the flipside, CYP3A4 inducers like carbamazepine, St. John's wort, phenytoin, or rifampin may reduce the concentration of alprazolam. Be aware that benzodiazepine withdrawal is risky and if a CYP3A4 inducer drops the concentration too much, you may see signs of withdrawal begin to precipitate. Anxiety, insomnia, twitching, tremors, and other CNS effects are possible. With benzodiazepines, abrupt withdrawal could also lead to seizure if severe enough. I think that is probably pretty unlikely with the initiation of a CYP3A4 inducer, but conceivable under the right circumstances.

Lorazepam avoids the CYP3A4 pathway which is definitely an advantage over alprazolam. If you have a patient that is taking a CYP3A4 inhibitor or inducer, it would be a strong consideration to use lorazepam versus alprazolam if a benzodiazepine is necessary. Clonazepam is also broken down by CYP3A4 and concentrations can be altered by having an inducer or inhibitor on board.

Propylene Glycol

In the metronidazole section, we discussed products that may have components that will interact with it. Medications containing propylene glycol can cause a disulfiram reaction when your patient is also receiving metronidazole. Some commonly used injectable or rectal benzodiazepine products that may contain propylene glycol include lorazepam and diazepam.

CYP2C19 Effects

Diazepam is a bit more complicated than lorazepam when it comes to drug interactions. CYP2C19 plays a role in the metabolism of diazepam. In addition to CYP2C19, CYP3A4 also plays a potential role in breaking down diazepam. A drug like fluconazole which can have significant 2C19 inhibition will be likely to raise the concentration of diazepam. Be on the lookout for enhanced effects from diazepam if agents that impact CYP3A4 or CYP2C19 are used.

CNS Depressant

Zolpidem is a relatively common agent used for the management of insomnia. As far as the majority of effects it can cause, I essentially lump it into the benzodiazepine category. Sedation, confusion, fall risk, and other CNS adverse effects can happen. All of the similar CNS depressant drug interactions that are associated with benzodiazepines apply to zolpidem.

CYP3A4

CYP3A4 is mostly responsible for the breakdown of zolpidem. This means that the use of CYP3A4 inhibitors or inducers is going to impact zolpidem concentrations. Pay attention to the risk of adverse effects when inhibitors are used, and lower concentrations when inducers are used.

Trazodone

CNS Depressant

Trazodone is used way more often for its sedative properties than for its antidepressant properties. A target dose of 200 mg or higher for depression is common. Most commonly you will see doses less than 200 mg used for the management of insomnia. Normally, we start with 25-50 mg at bedtime. As you can imagine, if we are using this medication for insomnia, it is sedating and has a CNS depressant type effect. All the CNS depressant drug interactions that apply to opioids and benzodiazepines would also apply to trazodone.

Serotonin Syndrome

Serotonergic activity is possible with the use of trazodone. While it is important to recognize this fact, the likelihood of trazodone inducing serotonin syndrome is very low. Even when other medications are on board, trazodone is typically used at low doses for its sedative effects. The lower the dose, the less likely we will need to worry about serotonin syndrome. I would possibly have a little more reservation if you have a patient on an unusually high dose of an SSRI or another agent that can precipitate this effect.

CYP3A4

CYP3A4 is the primary mode of metabolism for trazodone. Any drug impacts on CYP3A4 can alter the concentration and potentially the risk for toxicity or ineffectiveness. Inducers would be likely to cause therapeutic failure while inhibitors of CYP3A4 would be more likely to lead to toxicity.

Bupropion

Seizure Risk

In any patient that has a history of seizures or is at risk for seizures, bupropion should generally be avoided. When I'm reviewing a patient's medication list, if I see an order for an antiepileptic agent, I also take a quick glance to ensure that the patient is not taking bupropion. Bupropion has the potential to lower the seizure threshold and increase the risk for seizures.

It is also advisable to review for other medications that can have additive seizure potential effects. Certain antipsychotics, tramadol, TCAs, and drugs for ADHD are a few common examples of medications that may be associated with lowering the seizure threshold and making a patient more susceptible to a seizure.

CYP2D6

One of the most well-known drug interactions with bupropion is its potential to inhibit CYP2D6. Because of this activity, I lump it into the same category as paroxetine and fluoxetine. Any interaction that paroxetine or fluoxetine has via CYP2D6, bupropion will likely have as well. Here's a case scenario demonstrating CYP2D6 inhibition with a TCA.

A 58 year old female has refractory depression and is managed by psychiatry. In addition to the depression, she has also had quite a bit of trouble with insomnia. She has been experiencing an increase in depressive symptoms and another agent is looking to be added to her regimen. She has had partial responses to many of her medications and is reluctant to come off of any of her current psych meds. Her current medication list includes:
- Nortriptyline 100 mg once daily
- Duloxetine 30 mg once daily
- Buspirone 10 mg BID

- Trazodone 100 mg at bedtime for sleep
- Aspirin 81 mg daily
- Lipitor 10 mg once daily
- Ibuprofen 400 mg three times per day

The primary provider adds bupropion extended-release 150 mg once daily for 7 days and then increase to 300 mg per day.

In 6 weeks, the patient is followed up with and notes to be feeling very lethargic, with complaints of dry mouth and a report of not being able to "think clearly".

In this situation, the likelihood of bupropion causing these side effects is low. These side effects definitely mimic the potential of anticholinergic effects. Bupropion can impact CYP2D6 which is a primary pathway for nortriptyline to be metabolized. Bupropion caused the drug levels of the nortriptyline to increase, leading to the potential adverse effects.

Looking back at this situation, the bupropion nortriptyline interaction should have been recognized prior to prescribing the bupropion. If it was deemed necessary that the bupropion was essential for the resolution of depression, a lower dose and more cautious approach should have been employed with closer monitoring of the patient. Alternatively, a preemptive dose reduction in nortriptyline could have been considered. Another possibility would be to check nortriptyline levels as this is often done anyway in the management of depression.

Dopamine Activity

While bupropion is considered an antidepressant, it is a bit different from other antidepressants in that it does not primarily impact serotonin. It is more likely to have dopaminergic activity. Because of this, it has the potential to have additive effects on dopamine agonist agents. Ropinirole, pramipexole, and carbidopa/levodopa toxicity and adverse effects may be more likely in patients who are taking bupropion in combination with any agent that has a net effect of increasing dopamine activity.

Metabolic Syndrome

Antipsychotics are well known to contribute to metabolic syndrome. Weight gain, hyperglycemia, and hyperlipidemia are all possible due to this risk. It is important to note that there are individual differences in the class of antipsychotics. The atypical (second generation) antipsychotics tend to have a stronger propensity to contribute to metabolic syndrome.

By contributing to metabolic syndrome, antipsychotics will directly oppose what we are trying to accomplish with the use of medications for diabetes and hypercholesterolemia. In the management of schizophrenia and bipolar disorder, it may absolutely be necessary to use an antipsychotic regardless of this risk. In a patient at risk for metabolic syndrome or who is taking medications for diabetes or hyperlipidemia, it would be important to avoid the highest risk agents. Clozapine and olanzapine are the two agents that have the highest potential to cause metabolic syndrome. Of the most commonly used antipsychotics, aripiprazole and ziprasidone tend to have the least impact on weight gain and metabolic syndrome.

QTc Prolongation

Similar to the metabolic syndrome risk, antipsychotics can have a cumulative risk for contributing to QTc prolongation. Also comparable to the risk for metabolic syndrome is the fact that some of the antipsychotics are more likely to contribute to this complication than others. Of the more commonly used agents, ziprasidone, risperidone, and quetiapine tend to be more likely to contribute to QTc prolongation. While aripiprazole still carries the precaution on QTc prolongation, it tends to be on the lower end of the risk spectrum.

Dopamine Antagonism

The primary mechanism through which antipsychotics work is through dopamine blockade. In psychosis and disorders that cause psychosis, it is theorized that there is a surplus of dopamine. By blocking dopamine in the brain we can help improve those symptoms. On the flipside, Parkinson's is a disease where there is a dopamine shortage.

Because antipsychotics essentially can blunt the effects of dopamine, this class of drugs can stifle the benefit from common Parkinson's medications like carbidopa/levodopa, ropinirole, and pramipexole. The typical antipsychotics like haloperidol are typically avoided due to their strong potential to block dopamine and increase the risk for extrapyramidal and pseudoparkinson's type symptoms.

Of the atypical antipsychotics, there is a continuum as to the degree that these agents can cause movement disorder side effects. Risperidone and paliperidone have stronger dopamine potential and would be more likely to counteract the effects of Parkinson's medications. Quetiapine, pimavanserin, and clozapine are least likely to blunt the effects of Parkinson's medications.

In addition to opposing effects, recall that there are some medications that are used for GI purposes that may have additive dopamine blocking effects. Prochlorperazine (Compazine) is classified as a first-generation antipsychotic because it has dopamine blocking activity. Even though it is classified as an antipsychotic, I still continue to see it occasionally for its use as an antiemetic. In addition to prochlorperazine, metoclopramide is another medication used in nausea and vomiting as well as gastroparesis that has significant dopamine blocking activity. Be aware of this increasing the risk of dopamine deficiency type adverse effects like extrapyramidal symptoms.

CNS Depressant

Sedation can happen with all of the antipsychotics but is more prominent with some versus others. Quetiapine and clozapine would be more likely to cause sedation and contribute to CNS depressant interactions. Aripiprazole and risperidone would be less likely to contribute to these interactions.

Anticholinergic Activity

Antipsychotics can contribute to anticholinergic burden which can be especially troublesome in our elderly population. Clozapine, olanzapine, and quetiapine tend to have a little higher risk for anticholinergic activity. Aripiprazole and ziprasidone are on the lower end of the spectrum of risk for additive anticholinergic activity.

Low Blood Pressure

Antipsychotics are definitely associated with hypotension. Be aware when a patient is reporting symptoms of low blood pressure like dizziness. In general, if blood pressure is too low, I'm going to likely review drugs specifically being used for hypertension first. If we can reduce those, that is typically my initial recommendation. Clozapine actually has this as a boxed warning. Be incredibly careful when titrating and restarting clozapine to ensure that we do it slowly enough to minimize this risk. Quetiapine is also fairly high on the risk scale for orthostatic hypotension. Aripiprazole tends to be on the lower-risk end of the spectrum.

Quetiapine

Because quetiapine is at least in part metabolized by CYP3A4, drugs that impact the function of this enzyme can alter the concentration and effectiveness of quetiapine. CYP3A4 inducers like carbamazepine and others can reduce the concentration of quetiapine. Strong CYP3A4 inhibitors like clarithromycin can reduce the metabolism of quetiapine which can increase the risk for adverse effects.

CYP1A2

Olanzapine and Clozapine are both impacted by CYP1A2. Any drug that induces CYP1A2 can lead to lower concentrations and risk for therapeutic failure. Any drug that inhibits CYP1A2 can increase the risk of toxicity. Here's a case scenario and drug interaction that you may have never thought about before.

A 28 year old male patient with schizophrenia is being treated with olanzapine 15 mg twice daily. He has been fairly well controlled and the dose has been stable for at least 6 months. His primary provider has been working with him to try to get him to stop smoking. He has not been smoking cigarettes for approximately 1 week. He is on varenicline to help with smoking cessation.

The patient is now reporting an increase in tremor and also feels very sedated. A CBC and thyroid function testing was done to help rule out the cause of the fatigue. Both were negative for any concerns. The PCP believed that the varenicline was the cause of the new-onset fatigue and tremor. Varenicline was stopped and the symptoms persisted.

I always recommend reviewing any type of change in a patient's routine. Changes in lifestyle, supplements, over-the-counter medications, or prescription medications can lead to new changes. In this scenario, stopping smoking allowed for the increased accumulation and side effects from the olanzapine. In schizophrenia, it is highly important to recognize that smoking changes can significantly alter concentrations of olanzapine and clozapine.

Olanzapine is broken down by CYP1A2. Smoking causes the induction of the CYP1A2 enzyme. The olanzapine smoking cessation interaction is one that we should educate our patients about. When CYP1A2 is inhibited, this would lead to higher concentrations of olanzapine. When CYP1A2 is induced, it would lead to a reduction in olanzapine concentrations.

CYP2D6

Risperidone is significantly metabolized by CYP2D6. Enzyme inducers or inhibitors could play a role in the metabolism of the drug. Corresponding antidepressants are sometimes used in combination with antipsychotics so recall that fluoxetine and paroxetine can inhibit CYP2D6 and increase the risk for risperidone adverse effects.

Aripiprazole

The breakdown of aripiprazole can be impacted by both CYP3A4 and CYP2D6. This can lead to a significant number of interactions that may alter the concentrations of aripiprazole. While there may be a lower risk for cumulative adverse effects like orthostasis, metabolic syndrome, and EPS compared to some of the other antipsychotics, there may be a higher likelihood of CYP enzyme interactions.

Serotonin and Norepinephrine Reuptake Inhibitors (SNRIs)

Norepinephrine Activity

Duloxetine and venlafaxine increase the activity of norepinephrine. As the dose of these drugs increases, we are more likely to have stronger norepinephrine effects. Norepinephrine is a neurotransmitter that can certainly increase blood pressure. In patients on medications to help manage their blood pressure, I definitely take a look to see if they are taking an SNRI. At low doses, I typically am not terribly concerned about this, but as doses of venlafaxine or duloxetine escalate, we are more likely to cause elevations in blood pressure which can directly oppose what we are trying to accomplish with antihypertensive therapy.

Serotonergic Activity

The two most commonly used SNRIs include venlafaxine (Effexor) and duloxetine (Cymbalta). Much like the SSRIs, SNRIs increase the amount of serotonin in the brain. Because of this, the risk for serotonin syndrome exists with this class. Virtually all of the potential serotonergic interactions that we discussed in the SSRI section will apply to the use of SNRIs. Here's a case example with a TCA and how the use of this combination should generally be avoided.

A 66-year-old female has a past medical history of diabetes, neuropathy, depression, and hypertension. In this case scenario, I discuss the use of a TCA with an SNRI. Her current medication list includes:

- Aspirin 81 mg daily
- Capsaicin cream PRN
- Amitriptyline 10 mg at night
- Metformin 500 mg BID
- Losartan 50 mg daily
- Glipizide 5 mg daily
- Duloxetine 30 mg daily

One of the first questions I would have in this case review is why would the patient be on the amitriptyline (TCA) with duloxetine (SNRI). I would dig into the patient history to try to figure out when and why these medications were added. I will say, that when I see TCAs dosed at night, it is often (at least in part) due to their sedative adverse effect. TCAs and SNRIs both inhibit the reuptake of serotonin and norepinephrine, so we do run the risk of duplicate effects. In general, I would try to avoid the TCA with an SNRI combination and in this situation, we may be able to easily titrate up on one and off of the other (again, this does depend upon what indication we are trying to use each of the agents for). In a 66-year-old, I'm not thrilled about the use of a TCA due to their potential anticholinergic effects.

I also want to point out in this case scenario, that duloxetine's inhibition of CYP2D6 may increase the concentrations of amitriptyline. This would further increase the risk for serotonin issues as well as the potential for amitriptyline adverse effects.

Antiplatelet Activity

Similar to the risk for serotonin syndrome, there is a theoretical risk for platelet inhibition. Also similar to the SSRIs, combinations of anticoagulants and antiplatelet agents with duloxetine or venlafaxine is ok in the majority of situations. Simply recognizing that the risk for bleeding may be elevated is important. Patient monitoring and education are going to be sufficient in the majority of cases. If you have a patient that has a low hemoglobin or is currently dealing with blood loss, a risk versus benefit assessment would be appropriate.

CYP2D6

Duloxetine and venlafaxine can both inhibit CYP2D6. While I would not consider the risk as significant as bupropion, paroxetine, or fluoxetine, it is important to recognize that it can increase concentrations of medications that rely on this pathway for metabolic breakdown. Tamoxifen is a medication that I always have in the back of my head when it comes to CYP2D6 because we would never want a situation where the potential effectiveness in cancer management is in doubt.

CYP1A2

Duloxetine does rely on the CYP1A2 pathway for the cessation of its physiological effects. Because this pathway is important in the metabolic breakdown of duloxetine, CYP1A2 inhibitors can alter concentrations in an upward fashion. Monitor your patient for adverse effects of duloxetine. Similar to olanzapine and clozapine, smoking tobacco products can induce the metabolism of duloxetine and potentially increase the risk of treatment failure. I wouldn't consider these combinations contraindicated with one another, so being aware and monitoring patients for clinical changes would be appropriate in the majority of situations.

CNS Stimulants

Additive Effects

Stimulants like methylphenidate, amphetamine salts, dextroamphetamine, and lisdexamfetamine are well known for their ability to cause elevations in blood pressure, heart rate, and other stimulant type effects. Pay attention to any medication added to a patient's regimen that may add on to this effect. Drugs like modafinil, caffeine, theophylline, and pseudoephedrine can all exacerbate some of the potential side effects of stimulants.

It is also important to keep an eye out for illicit drug use as well. Cocaine is a notorious stimulant that can exacerbate tachycardia, hypertension, and other stimulant type effects when used in combination with traditional prescription stimulants.

Opposing Effects

Stimulants do what the name of their class indicates. They can stimulate the central nervous system. While this can have its perks, pun intended, I have seen numerous cases where these drugs can impact other medications. If a patient has hypertension or a history of atrial fibrillation and is being managed with medication therapy for either of these issues, stimulants can create the exact opposite effect.

In addition to the cardiovascular risks, you need to be aware that stimulants can oppose the benefits of many psychotropic medications. Particularly, drugs used to help manage anxiety or insomnia can have their effectiveness reduced by adding a stimulant to a patient's medication regimen.

MAOI

Drugs with MAOI activity can have the risk of a tyramine reaction which can substantially raise blood pressure. If a patient is taking a medication with MAOI activity in combination with a stimulant, there is a significant concern for a hypertensive urgency or even emergency. It would be best to avoid this combination, but if they happen to be used together, we must carefully monitor vital signs and educate our patients about the potential risks.

Methylphenidate

Alcohol use with methylphenidate is not recommended. Alcohol can inhibit one of the mechanisms that methylphenidate is broken down by. Because of the inhibition of breakdown, the patient will have a higher risk for methylphenidate toxicity and adverse effects.

Tricyclic Antidepressants

Anticholinergic Activity

Commonly used tricyclic antidepressants include amitriptyline (Elavil) and nortriptyline (Pamelor). They are highly anticholinergic which limits their use compared to the much more tolerable SSRIs. The significant amount of anticholinergic activity associated with these drugs is one of the primary reasons they are listed in the Beers criteria.

All of the anticholinergic drug interactions that were discussed in the antihistamine section would apply to the tricyclics.

Gastroparesis can be a serious problem where the GI tract literally "slows down". This issue is common in patients with diabetes. Bloating, abdominal pain, nausea, vomiting, and a feeling of fullness are all possible symptoms of gastroparesis. There are also medications like anticholinergics that can worsen gastroparesis. Here's a case scenario where the anticholinergic effects from amitriptyline can combat the prokinetic effects of metoclopramide.

KD is a 62 year old female who has been having a lot of GI complaints. She often feels nauseous and does occasionally vomit. Her past medical history includes:
- diabetes
- gastroparesis
- osteoarthritis
- neuropathy
- depression

Her current medications include:
- metformin
- amitriptyline
- metoclopramide
- glipizide
- gabapentin
- acetaminophen

In this scenario, I would strongly look at what dose of amitriptyline this patient is taking. In addition, I would want to know what the patient is taking it for. I would suspect that amitriptyline is being used for depression and neuropathy.

Tri-cyclic antidepressants are one of many medication classes that are highly anticholinergic. Drugs with anticholinergic effects can "slow down" the GI tract which could obviously be a problem in this case. This could directly oppose any beneficial prokinetic effects from the metoclopramide. Finding an alternative to amitriptyline would be helpful to reduce the risk of exacerbating gastroparesis symptoms. If we are treating depression, an SSRI would be a preferred option. Alternatively, if amitriptyline is being used for pain and neuropathy type symptoms, an SNRI, or possibly increasing the gabapentin would be potential considerations.

QTc Prolongation

The tricyclics are associated with QTc prolongation. As a healthcare professional, we must recognize the cumulative risk and the importance of identifying risk factors, obtaining baseline EKG measurements, and minimizing the risk for using multiple agents that can prolong the QT interval. You can find further discussion on this in the amiodarone section.

CNS Depressant

The sedative properties of tricyclic antidepressants are often taken advantage of to help out our patients. While they have a somewhat overlapping mechanism of action compared with the SNRIs, they are much more anticholinergic and sedating. In a patient that has fibromyalgia and has difficulty with insomnia, a TCA may be a more appropriate choice to help with insomnia and fibromyalgia compared to an SNRI like duloxetine. With the reward also comes the risk of over sedating the patient or having future medications added that can cause excessive sedation which can be undesirable and unsafe. We discussed numerous other agents in the opioid section that can have additive CNS depressant effects.

CYP2D6

Both amitriptyline and nortriptyline primarily depend upon CYP2D6 for metabolic breakdown. Because of this, any drug that inhibits CYP2D6 is likely to raise concentrations of these two TCAs. Monitor for an increased risk of adverse effects like dry mouth, confusion, sedation, urinary retention, and constipation.

Serotonin Risks

Drug interactions regarding serotonin exist with tricyclic antidepressants. The mechanism of action for TCAs overlaps with SNRIs so any drug interactions that may occur as a consequence of higher serotonin levels can occur due to the use of TCAs. Review the section on SSRIs for details on more common agents that can affect serotonin. For the overwhelming majority of patients, we would almost never use a TCA like amitriptyline or nortriptyline in combination with an SNRI or SSRI.

There is one definite exception that you may see with this recommendation. In a patient who is taking a large dose of an SSRI, we may enlist a cross-taper strategy if we wanted to try that patient on a TCA. This is to help avoid the risk of discontinuation syndrome. Abruptly discontinuing moderate to high doses of antidepressants can lead to insomnia, anxiety, stomach upset, and other CNS changes.

I want to outline some clinical common sense in the scenario below and also help you understand that different public drug interaction programs may flag different interactions. In the situation below, I looked up amitriptyline and tramadol on Medscape and Drugs.com.

Medscape and Drugs.com both report different interactions on this one. Medscape reports to monitor for increased serotonin levels as well as to look out for both of these medications having sedative properties. Drugs.com, which I tend to trust a little less, says we should be concerned about monitoring for seizures.

This is the really frustrating part about drug interactions. Many times there isn't guidance about the severity and, if there is, the severity may differ depending upon the program you are using. So, here is my thought process when looking at interactions like this one with conflicting data;

- Has the patient been taking and tolerating these meds for a while or is it a new start?
- Are both medications absolutely necessary and/or what alternatives exist?
- Does the patient already have a diagnosis that might make this interaction worse (i.e. are you starting tramadol in a patient that already has seizures)?
- How solid is the evidence that the drug interaction program is using or how many case reports exist?
- Review the dosing of each medication. Is the patient being started on a moderate to high dose? Maybe they shouldn't be if we are concerned about an interaction.
- Anticipate problems and educate the patient about what outcomes or adverse effects may be anticipated from a potential drug interaction.

CYP3A4

Buspirone is primarily used for the management of anxiety disorders. I have also rarely seen it used for augmentation in depression. In general, the risk of clinically significant drug interactions is fairly low. Benzodiazepines would typically be considered a much riskier agent.

It is primarily broken down by CYP3A4 and like with many other agents, alterations in the activity of CYP3A4 can lead to alterations in blood levels of the drug. CYP3A4 inhibitors are likely to cause elevations in concentrations and increase the risk for toxicity. CYP3A4 inducers have the potential to lower concentrations and cause treatment failure.

Serotonin Activity

Buspirone does have modest serotonin activity but can be used in combination with other serotonergic agents such as SSRIs, TCAs, SNRIs, or MAOIs. Simply monitoring for the risk of serotonin syndrome would be appropriate. Much like with other serotonergic interactions, paying attention to the serotonergic burden is important. Patients who are receiving high dose MAOIs or SSRIs will certainly be at greater risk for serotonin syndrome occurring versus those taking low doses.

Sedation

Buspirone can cause some mild sedation. When comparing it to another anti-anxiety agent, lorazepam, or other benzodiazepines, buspirone is much more benign. Benzodiazepines will have a much greater potential to cause CNS depression and sedation compared to buspirone. This is especially true in the elderly population.

Mirtazapine

Sedation

Mirtazapine is significantly sedating as it does have some antihistamine effects. Because of this fact, it is often utilized in the management of insomnia. It can also have additive effects if a patient is taking other CNS depressant medications. Interestingly, mirtazapine also has noradrenergic activity which causes stimulation. The noradrenergic activity is more likely to happen as the dose escalates.

In a patient that is overly sedated, I can't say I would likely recommend increasing the dose of mirtazapine for fear of not knowing exactly where that sweet spot is for the patient. I would be more likely to recommend discontinuing mirtazapine if there were no other purpose for the medication other than the management of insomnia.

Serotonin Increases

While not by the traditional SSRI method or likely to the extent of SSRIs, mirtazapine can potentially raise levels of serotonin. Because of this, we do still need to pay attention to the serotonergic load and ultimately the risk for serotonin syndrome.

CYP Enzymes

As with many drugs, multiple CYP enzymes play a role in the metabolism of mirtazapine. CYP3A4 and CYP1A2 are the two major players that are likely to have clinically significant impacts. Being aware of patients who start medications that impact either of these pathways is important because mirtazapine concentrations could be affected. Drugs that affect these pathways typically aren't going to be contraindicated, but the risk for clinically significant alterations in concentrations is possible.

MAOIs

Tyramine Foods

The most commonly used MAOI I have seen used in the management of depression is tranylcypromine (Parnate). One of the biggest concerns with MAOIs are dietary restrictions. It makes this a very messy drug. Tyramine is a compound that is found in various foods. Monoamine oxidase found in the digestive tract breaks down this compound. By inhibiting these enzymes, a significant and unusual amount of tyramine may get into the systemic circulation. Tyramine can be commonly found in aged cheeses, smoked fish and other meats, and certain beers. Many patients I know enjoy eating those items once in a while. If enough tyramine containing food is consumed, the accumulation in the systemic circulation can escalate. Excessive tyramine can substantially raise blood pressure and put a patient into a hypertensive crisis.

Hypertension

Because of the tyramine reaction, many drugs that raise blood pressure will be contraindicated with the use of MAOIs. Stimulants like methylphenidate should be avoided in combination. MAOIs are a class of medication that only a specialist is likely to use, but one that you have to be aware of because it's more than likely that any agent you want to add to a patient's regimen will have a high likelihood of interacting with it.

Serotonin

MAOIs are used very seldom, and one of the biggest reasons is the number of drugs that are contraindicated with its use. Many of those contraindicated interactions have to do with how MAOIs can increase serotonin levels. The use of many of the traditional antidepressants with an MAOI is contraindicated due to serotonin syndrome risks. Avoidance of SSRIs, SNRIs, mirtazapine, and TCAs is recommended when a patient is taking an MAOI. The overwhelming majority of agents that can raise serotonin levels that were discussed in the SSRI section are going to be contraindicated with the use of MAOIs. MAOIs are another class of medication that alerts me to look at a drug interaction profile prior to recommending any changes in a patient's medication regimen.

Anticholinergic

To add to all of the other risks mentioned with MAOIs, they can also have anticholinergic activity. Be aware of the anticholinergic burden and the risk for anticholinergic adverse effects when an MAOI is added to a patient's medication list.

With the use of beta-agonists that are administered via the respiratory route, there are really very few clinically significant drug interactions. For most of these agents, systemic absorption is minimal to none. With that said, be aware of patients who may be taking large amounts or frequently using these medications. Common beta-agonists include the short-acting agents such as albuterol and levalbuterol. Commonly used longer-acting beta-agonists include formoterol, arformoterol, vilanterol, indacaterol, and salmeterol. Here are a few common interactions that may come up in clinical practice.

Beta-Blockers

Any beta-blocker can inhibit the function of beta receptors. Many beta-blockers are "cardioselective", which means that they primarily block the Beta-1 receptors on the heart. It is important to remember that even "cardioselectivity" will go away as drug concentrations increase. The albuterol beta-blocker interaction is real and is significant. Let's discuss how significant it is and what questions you should ask yourself.

The very first question I would assess is which beta-blocker are we talking about as not all beta-blockers are created equally! It is critical to remember that non-selective beta-blockers will have a much greater impact on beta-2 receptors. Common examples of non-selective beta-blockers include propranolol, timolol, and nadolol.

Is the drug necessary and what are we treating are two straightforward questions to consider before initiating albuterol. Nearly 100% of the time, breathing and managing an acute breathing exacerbation is going to be a top priority. That leaves us with the beta-blocker and identifying what we are treating with that medication. If we are treating hypertension, migraines, or tremors, these would all be good examples where alternatives exist and the risk of switching to something different is typically not going to be life-threatening.

Remember that beta-blocking effects are generally going to be dose-dependent. The higher the dose, the more likely that we are going to cause respiratory problems and increase the significance of the albuterol beta-blocker interaction. With nearly all medications that have receptor selectivity, it is also true that as the dose rises, selectivity starts to decline.

If the beta-blocker is absolutely necessary, I would definitely want to make sure we could use a beta-1 selective agent if at all possible. The stronger the inhibitory effects that we have on beta-2 receptors, the more likely our albuterol effects will be marginalized.

With many drug interactions, sometimes the best we can do is monitor the patient over the course of time and continue to weigh the risks versus the benefits. If you identify a patient that has been to the emergency department twice in the last two months for breathing-related difficulties and the patient remains on propranolol 80 mg BID, you need to address this situation and recognize that propranolol is likely contributing to this situation.

If a patient remains on metoprolol and a beta-agonist for years without issue, we can probably use this combination indefinitely and continue to assess and monitor the patient's respiratory status.

Here's a case scenario that demonstrates the risk with non-selective beta-blockers in patients who may be at risk for respiratory distress.

A 78 year old female has had difficulty with essential tremor. She has had the tremor most of her life and has managed with primidone. The primidone has been well tolerated. She is now recently reporting that the primidone doesn't seem to be working as well as it used to and is wondering what can be done.

The primary care provider initiates propranolol 20 mg three times per day. This is not effective so the provider gradually increases the dose to 60 mg three times daily. The 78 year old reports tolerating the dose without dropping the blood pressure and pulse too low, but is reporting a new symptom of difficulty breathing. She had apparently had some asthma as a child which had not been an issue as an adult.

Important things to remember with this effect on the lungs is that selectivity of agents is important. Beta-1 selective medications are typically less likely to cause this effect on the lungs. Unfortunately in this situation, the beta-1 selective medications typically aren't as effective as propranolol. The other thing to remember is that as we escalate the dose, we are more likely to lose selectivity as well as cause adverse effects.

The patient and provider elected to taper back and off of the propranolol and stick with the primidone alone.

Tachycardia and QTc prolongation

Albuterol and other beta-agonists can have dose-dependent increases on tachycardia and QTc prolongation. If the patient takes one or two puffs of albuterol once a month, this is likely not going to cause an issue. With that said, I think it is important to look at other agents that may be contributing to tachycardia or QTc prolongation and assess if they are still necessary or could possibly be reduced.

Medications like antipsychotics, ondansetron, macrolides, quinolones, and others could have the potential to be discontinued in many situations. Reviewing the appropriateness of long term use of these agents is one of my first steps in addressing QTc prolongation. Antibiotics and anti-nausea medications that contribute to QTc prolongation are hopefully only necessary for short periods of time so that should be helpful.

As far as tachycardia goes, it is important to recognize that many stimulants or other drugs that can stimulate beta receptors can have additive effects and exacerbate tachycardia. Stimulants like methylphenidate and amphetamine derivatives can cause tachycardia on their own but could have additive effects if albuterol was frequently or excessively used. Mirabegron is a beta-3 agonist that can be used in the setting of urinary frequency. This is another example of a medication where if the dose was increased, selectivity for beta-3 receptors could go down and increase the risk of beta-1 activation and tachycardia.

One mistake I have seen patients and providers make is not recognizing the class of medication that the patient is using. One example I remember encountering is a COPD patient who was taking formoterol routinely as their long-acting beta-agonist. In addition to this, the patient would take their albuterol inhaler with "Duonebs". Remember that Duonebs contains albuterol in combination with ipratropium. This higher level of intake of beta-agonists would be much more likely to contribute to cardiac complications than simply taking one of these agents at a time.

Hypokalemia

Systemic beta-agonists can have impacts on electrolytes. The most concerning impact would be on potassium levels. Albuterol and other

221

beta-2 agonists can contribute to hypokalemia. The likelihood of this happening when beta-2 agonists are inhaled is extremely low. However, it might be advisable to keep an eye out for this in patients who use large amounts of beta-agonists and who may be at risk for hypokalemia. Those patients who may be at higher risk for hypokalemia include those who have a past history of hypokalemia or who are taking loop or thiazide diuretics that can cause depletion of potassium on their own.

Inhaled Anticholinergics

Similar to the beta-agonists, there are long-acting and short-acting anticholinergic agents. While you will often see many drug interactions flag with these agents, you must recognize that the percentage of drug that gets into systemic circulation is typically going to be low. The traditional systemic anticholinergic adverse effects will depend upon the percentage of systemic absorption.

Additive Anticholinergic Effects

The likelihood of additive anticholinergic effects strictly depends upon the amount used and the percentage that is bioavailable. Ipratropium, tiotropium, aclidinium, glycopyrrolate, and umeclidinium will not typically be absorbed systemically to a significant extent to be a problem. If anticholinergic signs and symptoms are overt, I would first look at other systemic agents that the patient is taking and reduce or discontinue those medications as appropriate. I would not target reducing respiratory anticholinergics unless it is an extreme situation or the inhaled anticholinergic seems unnecessary for some reason.

With that stated, there is one really bothersome adverse effect that tends to come up specifically with the inhaled anticholinergics. Because we are orally inhaling these medications, it makes sense that a significant number of patients might report dry mouth. We will likely need the anticholinergic for managing COPD and the nuisance of dry mouth would not necessitate the discontinuation of a long-acting anticholinergic. Reports of dry mouth would, however, prompt me to investigate the patient's entire anticholinergic burden. I've often found that many patients who report dry mouth are also experiencing other anticholinergic adverse effects like constipation, urinary retention, etc. Assessment of systemic anticholinergic agents with possible reduction or discontinuation would be my first step in trying to reduce dry mouth symptoms. We can manage the adverse effect of dry mouth by increasing fluid intake or consider a saliva substitute.

Caution With Drug Interaction Programs

When you run a drug interaction check on a patient's inhaled anticholinergics, it will often incorporate and associate anticholinergic risk for all oral, inhaled, and systemic anticholinergic interactions. One example of this is ipratropium opposing the efficacy of acetylcholinesterase inhibitors. Ipratropium's systemic absorption is less than 10%. The clinical significance of this interaction is likely negligible. Similar to this interaction is the risk for GI ulceration due to potassium supplements getting stuck in the GI tract. Recall that anticholinergics slow down the GI tract and could increase the risk of potassium tablets or capsules getting stuck in the esophagus or other GI locations. Ipratropium's effect on the GI tract is likely negligible due to the very low systemic absorption.

Inhaled Corticosteroids

CYP3A4

Systemic absorption of corticosteroids is likely going to be more concerning to your patients. This may be particularly true in the setting of pediatrics. It is important to recognize that fluticasone is broken down by CYP3A4. The stronger the inhibitor of CYP3A4, the more likely we are to have clinically significant systemic concentrations. As systemic concentrations rise, the risk for HPA suppression and all of the other negative adverse effects rises as well. In addition to HPA suppression, osteoporosis and hyperglycemia are commonly associated risks. One unique aspect of this interaction is that fluticasone comes in different formulations. The risk of this interaction having clinically significant impacts is greater if we are using fluticasone propionate (Flovent) compared to fluticasone furoate (in combination with vilanterol as Breo Ellipta).

This leads to the question as to what we should do about this risk. After all, inhaled corticosteroids are a mainstay of treatment in asthma. Avoiding drugs that inhibit CYP3A4 or at least minimizing the duration of their use would be my first step. If a CYP3A4 inhibitor is necessary long term, I'd review the use of the fluticasone. If the patient's asthma is controlled, a reduction of the inhaled corticosteroid might be considered. Another potential alternative would be to consider fluticasone furoate which may have a lower risk as mentioned above. Lastly, we'd want to monitor these patients for potential systemic adverse effects of corticosteroids. Hyperglycemia, HPA suppression, and osteoporosis risk would all be potential concerns.

Immunosuppression

Systemic corticosteroids can increase the risk of immunosuppression. This is especially true in patients who are taking other medications that may suppress the immune system. But what about the inhaled corticosteroids? This all goes back to the amount absorbed and in the systemic circulation. The risk for immunosuppression is not something I worry about much. Patients taking other immunosuppressives are likely to be followed by a specialist. The risk for infection is something we should be monitoring and tracking in any patient taking an immunosuppressive drug.

One addendum that I wanted to add here is the risk of thrush. Inhaled corticosteroids are notorious for being associated with contributing to thrush. Rinsing the mouth following administration is critical and is something that we want to ensure is being done. Patients on immunosuppressive therapy in addition to their inhaled corticosteroids may be at even higher risk for this complication.

Roflumilast

CYP3A4 Impact

Roflumilast is occasionally used in the setting of COPD. It is broken down by CYP3A4 so inducers of this enzyme will reduce concentrations and inhibitors will increase roflumilast concentrations. If a CYP3A4 inhibitor is utilized, we would simply monitor for the risk of adverse effects. Commonly associated side effects with the use of roflumilast include psychiatric changes like anxiety, insomnia, and depression. In addition, weight loss can be a problem with roflumilast.

CYP1A2 Impact

To a lesser extent, roflumilast is also metabolized by CYP1A2. Drugs that inhibit this metabolic pathway could increase the concentrations of roflumilast. The likelihood of this being clinically significant is less than the probability of CYP3A4 alterations having a meaningful impact.

Enzyme Inducers

One of the most concerning and critical interactions with oral contraceptives from a patient perspective is the risk for contraceptive failure. Classic enzyme inducers can lower concentrations of ethinyl estradiol and possibly norethindrone. Carbamazepine, phenytoin, rifampin, oxcarbazepine, St. John's wort, and phenobarbital are all classic examples of enzyme inducers that can reduce the effectiveness of birth control and leave our patient at risk for pregnancy. In the neurology section, I provided an example of another medication, topiramate, that can increase the risk for pregnancy. Here's another case example:

A 32 year old female has been struggling with fatigue, sadness, and overall symptoms of depression. Rather than utilizing traditional antidepressants as recommended by her primary care provider, the patient had heard from a friend that the herbal supplement St. John's Wort had helped with their symptoms so she decided to give it a try. Three months later, the patient was experiencing fatigue and had not had her normal monthly cycle. She took a pregnancy test and found out she indeed was expecting even though she had been taking her Ortho-Tri-Cyclen (birth control) as prescribed. What happened? We can never 100% say, but St. John's Wort does have the potential to reduce the effectiveness of birth control, making an unexpected pregnancy more likely. St. John's Wort is a notorious herbal supplement that can interact with many prescription medications (cholesterol meds, seizure meds, Coumadin etc.). Even though there is easy access to herbal supplements and over-the-counter (OTCs) medications it does not always mean they are safe.

Cigarette Smoking

There are some risks associated with the use of birth control. There is a boxed warning with regard to cigarette smoking. Patients taking oral contraceptives who are smokers and over the age of 35 are at an increased risk for cardiovascular events. The additive effects of oral contraceptives in combination with the cardiovascular risks associated with smoking put our patients in this category at a big risk for problems like heart attack and stroke. Finding other means of contraception would be critical. Alternatively, encouraging and convincing our patients to quit smoking would be an awesome victory in patient care. This is ideal. A progesterone-only option would be considered safer than combination contraception.

Antiestrogen Therapy

Antiestrogens can be used in the management of estrogen receptor-positive breast cancer. Anastrozole is a good example of this type of medication. From a mechanism of action standpoint, drugs like anastrozole ultimately reduce the production of estrogen. By giving estrogen we are essentially providing the body more of the hormone that is contributing to cancer growth. As you can imagine, this is not a good thing and should be avoided.

Absorption

Just as problematic as an enzyme inducer, drugs that block or blunt absorption of oral contraceptives can increase the risk for pregnancy. Reduced concentrations of ethinyl estradiol and norethindrone can cause treatment failure. Cholestyramine is a classic example of a drug that can block the absorption and potentially lead to this issue. Here's a case scenario.

KM is a 38 year old female who is taking ethinyl estradiol and norethindrone for oral contraceptive purposes. She has a history of irritable bowel syndrome. She has been taking loperamide but doesn't feel that it has been helping with her diarrhea. She would like an alternative agent.

Her primary care provider prescribes colestipol. Colestipol is a bile acid sequestrant that I have seen used off-label in clinical practice for its potential to help with diarrhea. She was instructed to take it once daily, but not instructed when to take it. She begins taking it every morning with her birth control and finds it moderately helpful.

Within the next few months, she discovers that she has become pregnant and wondered why and how this could have happened. Because colestipol has the potential to bind to oral contraceptives, it could have played a role in reducing concentrations and contributing to her pregnancy.

Alteration of Thyroid Replacement

There is some modest evidence that estrogen therapy could alter thyroid replacement. I would not put this high on my scale of severe drug interactions. This can be pretty easily managed and accounted for by monitoring TSH.

Alteration of Blood Sugar

There is some evidence that using birth control can cause alterations in blood sugar. More specifically, it would be most likely to produce a modest increase in blood sugars. This is not something that I would consider a strong effect. In patients who have diabetes and are a taking medications for it, it could have a minor opposition type effect. Generally, nothing but monitoring is going to be necessary for this interaction. Obviously, if you notice that a patient's blood sugars have been elevated substantially from this effect, you might consider the risk versus benefit of reducing the oral contraceptive dose or consider trying an alternative method of birth control.

Norethindrone (Minipill, POP)

Enzyme Inducers

Progesterone only pills (POPs) will have many similar drug interactions to traditional, combination birth control. Enzyme inducers are no exception and can cause the same problem with this type of birth control. Treatment failure is a real possibility if norethindrone is given in combination with an enzyme inducer.

Bile Acid Sequestrants

Also similar to traditional oral contraceptives is the risk for norethindrone concentrations to be reduced by bile acid sequestrants like cholestyramine and colestipol. This mechanism is the same as it is for oral contraceptives. Altering the timing of administration or avoiding the use of this type of agent would be the most important strategy to mitigate this interaction.

Medroxyprogesterone (Depo-Provera)

Enzyme Inducers

Much like norethindrone, medroxyprogesterone is a progesterone-only medication. Depo-Provera is the brand name of the most commonly used long-acting injection of this agent. The enzyme induction interaction still applies to this medication much like it does with norethindrone and combination oral contraceptives.

Nitrate Interaction

Avoidance of nitrates in combination with phosphodiesterase-5 inhibitors is recommended. The risk of this interaction is substantial hypotension. I discussed this interaction in more detail when I discussed the use of nitrates in the cardiovascular section.

Blood Pressure Lowering Medications

Interestingly, sildenafil was originally created to be a medication that lowers blood pressure. In the clinical trials, it was found that males were reporting that they were experiencing erections. Because of this discovery, the company that made sildenafil began to look at its potential to treat erectile dysfunction. It ultimately received approval for the indication of erectile dysfunction. However, its blood pressure-lowering potential should be noted. If you have patients that are susceptible to low blood pressure or are being managed on antihypertensives, sildenafil and the other PDE-5 inhibitors can have an additive effect.

The most likely initial management strategy will be to assess blood pressure and educate our patients about the risk of dizziness, falls, and syncope due to low blood pressure. In the event that our patient is experiencing these issues, it is important to reassess the dose of the PDE-5 inhibitor as well as our current antihypertensive regimen. In the setting of unacceptable hypotension, dose reductions would be appropriate.

Alpha-Blockers

Alpha-blockers can be considered antihypertensive, but can also be used in the setting of BPH. They can raise the risk of hypotension. In patients who are taking an alpha-blocker for BPH, be able to recognize the importance of selectivity. Tamsulosin may be a more appropriate choice if patients are at risk for hypotension or have a past history of experiencing this adverse effect. This may be especially true in a patient taking a PDE-5 inhibitor.

CYP3A4 Inhibition

Sildenafil is broken down in part by CYP3A4. By inhibiting this enzyme, we run the risk of higher sildenafil concentrations. Hypotension is a concentration-dependent effect and would be more likely to occur if a CYP3A4 inhibitor was added to a patients' regimen. Similar to the interaction with antihypertensives, monitoring for hypotension and dose reduction(s) might be considered. In addition to the risk for hypotension, flushing, headache, and stomach upset might be possible adverse effects to be aware of.

5-Alpha-Reductase Inhibitors

Opposition of Beneficial Effects

I had an elderly male patient recently started on midodrine due to orthostasis. Midodrine is an alpha agonist. He was not receiving any other medications that would be likely to lower blood pressure. This patient had a history of BPH and was not currently on medication for this indication. The primary provider noted worsening symptoms of retention following the addition of midodrine and added Proscar (finasteride) to help manage the symptoms.

As you could imagine, the patient wasn't very happy with this as finasteride is a 5-alpha reductase inhibitor used to shrink the prostate. Shrinking the prostate with the use of this medication takes weeks to months. The patient experienced no acute benefit.

With this brief scenario, I wanted to create two very important educational points.

Midodrine is an alpha agonist and if we think about this mechanism of action, it directly opposes the action of alpha-blockers as well as 5-alpha reductase inhibitors. In this situation, an alpha-blocker would have been useful for acute symptoms of retention but would be likely to exacerbate the hypotension.

Lesson number two is a mistake I've seen a few times. The thought that Proscar or other 5-alpha reductase inhibitors (Avodart – dutasteride) will treat BPH in the short term. As above, these drugs take a long time to work and are not going to provide relief in the short term.

An alternative option in this case, would be fludrocortisone for orthostasis. This medication (corticosteroid) certainly has plenty of clinical quirks as well, so digging into the patient history would be critically important.

Opposition of Adverse Effects

5-alpha-reductase inhibitors, like finasteride, reduce testosterone effects. Because of this, one of the major adverse effects includes sexual dysfunction. This can directly oppose the beneficial effects of agents that are used to manage sexual dysfunction. Finasteride adverse effects can oppose the benefits of medications like the PDE-5 inhibitors.

Tamoxifen

CYP2D6 Inhibitors

We've discussed this interaction at length, but I want to make sure this is in here for completeness. Any medication that can inhibit the action of CYP2D6 has the potential to lower concentrations of tamoxifen's active metabolite. This can ultimately reduce the effectiveness of tamoxifen as an agent in breast cancer. Common examples of medications that can inhibit CYP2D6 include paroxetine, fluoxetine, bupropion, mirabegron, and duloxetine.

Warfarin

This is a bit of a complex drug interaction and happens on two different levels. Initially, when I think of tamoxifen, I recall that it can cause blood clots as part of its adverse effect profile. This can negatively impact the beneficial effects of anticoagulation. This is true regardless of the anticoagulant that is being used.

Specific to warfarin is the fact that tamoxifen has the potential to inhibit CYP2C9. If you recall from metronidazole and Bactrim, inhibition of CYP2C9 can lead to substantial increases in INR. In this situation, we are probably more likely to transition warfarin to a newer anticoagulant if there is evidence to support an alternative. A risk-benefit assessment of tamoxifen should also be done with the oncology specialist involved in the patient's care. If the patient has experienced a DVT while taking tamoxifen, alternative therapy may be considered.

Because of both these potential interactions, this presents a very challenging situation where communication between specialty and primary care is critical.

CYP3A4 Inducers

This interaction is considered controversial at this point in time, but in my opinion, it would be best to avoid using any CYP3A4 inducers in combination with tamoxifen. CYP3A4 is involved in the metabolic breakdown and potentially activation of tamoxifen and its active metabolites. It appears that the net effect may be a reduction in effectiveness and because of this, it is probably advisable to try to avoid classic enzyme inducers like phenytoin and carbamazepine.

If you found this book helpful, I'd be so appreciative if you'd leave a review on Amazon! Thank you in advance!

If you have any feedback on this book or suggestions for future educational materials, shoot me an email at mededucation101@gmail.com

Also be sure to take advantage of the free resources at Meded101.com and RealLifePharmacology.com

For our entire list of premium content, checkout meded101.com/store

Made in the USA
Las Vegas, NV
24 August 2023

76567560R00128